Can You Come Here Where I Am?

The Poetry and Prose of
Seven Breast Cancer Survivors

Can You Come Here Where I Am?

The Poetry and Prose of
Seven Breast Cancer Survivors

By The Write-Away Group

Rita Busch

Judy Thibault Klevins

Daena Kluegel

Jana Morgana

Helen Rash

Katherine Traynham

Lesley Tyson

E.M. Press, Inc.
Manassas, VA

ISBN: 1-880664-25-9
Library of Congress Catalog Card Number: 98-14173

E. M. Press, Inc.
P.O. Box 4057
Manassas, VA 20108

to Helen, with love

ACKNOWLEDGMENTS

We have so many people to thank, it would be another book in itself, so we can excuse ourselves because it would be like too many guests at a very small wedding. But there are two people we owe even more than the usual thank-yous for support and encouragement that friends and family have offered.

Marcy Heidish is an award-winning author of six novels including *A Woman Called Moses*, the story of Harriet Tubman, which also became a TV movie. She offered to lead a writing group for breast cancer survivors in the fall of 1995 and continued long after funding for her grant ran out. She's served as chaplain in jails, nursing homes, hospitals, and among the homeless and has trained volunteer ministers in pastoral care. Her most recent book, *Who cares? Simple Ways YOU Can Reach Out*, addresses specific ways to practice the art of caring and the unique situations facing care-givers of those with AIDS, depression, or suicidal behavior. She began our workshop by bringing us an antique quilt, showing us how hundreds of individual pieces added in no discernible pattern could end up as something so beautiful. And one night, she said, "I think you could have a book." We hope she'll think we've made something beautiful out of these pieces of ourselves.

Kathy Dorner, Coordinator of The Cancer Center at Columbia-Arlington Hospital, has done everything *except* write this book herself. She offered the space for the group to meet, fed us, held our hands, did our mailings, brought us more people, promoted our work—all in addition to her social work, counseling, and administration of The Cancer Center. Did we mention she has a wonderful husband and two sons, one grown and one nearly? She is the person you hope to meet when you walk into a hospital: tireless, deeply caring, and committed to making medicine intersect with humanity in a compassionate way. She is irreplaceable, and we aren't the only ones who know it. Kathy, this is your work, too. You always remind us that you don't *really* know what it's like, since you haven't (Thank Heaven) had breast cancer yourself. You can quit saying that now. It's very clear to us that you "get it."

CONTENTS

Bungee-Jumping Into The Treatment Abyss

You made decisions you don't like, you're doing the best you can, you want to be really brave some days and others, you want to jump off a bridge. No matter how you prepare, the reality of treatment is different for every woman. It may be harder or easier than you expect, but it's yours alone and so you grit your teeth and do it. You may lose your hair, you don't look like yourself, you're fighting like crazy for something that's "Normal"—meaning, "Not about cancer." And you do it. You want to live.

It's Over Already?

Take a deep breath. At first, you can only think about starting treatment. Then you put your head down and push to just get through treatment. Before you know it, the period you were sure would seem like "forever" is over. And when the dust settles, you have to put yourself back together—again.

It's Never Over, Is It?

You lived through treatment, you've made the hard decisions, you've lost some friends and gained others, found out how strong you are or how strong your family is. And now, no one's looking for cancer in your body anymore—except you. There will be check-ups but, in between, how do you start to "get over" what happened? Can you?

Millions Of Us

It's a terrible sorority to join, but we're not alone. Sooner or later, you'll realize you're living again—after cancer. Some can do it in the middle of treatment and some not until years later. But you'll have joy, despite the side road you were forced onto. There will still be fear from time to time, but it seems manageable most of the time. And so you go on from here.

You're changed. Never the same. Some people say, in a crisis, you only become more of what you already are. Others insist the only real change in people is almost always the result of a dramatic crisis. Eleanor Roosevelt said women were like tea bags—you didn't know how strong they were until they were in hot water. Life is funny—the women we know who've fought breast cancer laugh more than women who've never had it. What could that be about?

Daena Kluegel
Kathe Traynham
Rita Busch
Lesley Tyson
Jana Morgana
Judy Thibault Klevins
Helen Rash

PROLOGUE

HELP ME
by Katherine Traynham

Everybody wants to help. Thank goodness. Everybody needs to help. The rare bird wants to be left alone to do it alone. Not me. I am always so pleased and so grateful when someone says, "Is there anything I can do?" and they seem to mean it. Yes, there's plenty you can do. Or not do.

Come Here Where I Am. The sweetest thing that happened to me when the news went around that I had breast cancer was that people called me. I didn't have to call many of them. I was afraid and angry. Most people were sad and kind. That was okay. The best reaction I got was the dear friend who called and said, "Oh, God! I am so pissed that you have this!" She ranted for a few minutes. Not at fate. Just at cancer. It felt wonderful for her to be where I was. I didn't want to have it. She didn't want me to have it. She could be where I was for a minute. Pissed.

Don't try to talk me out of what I feel. Don't try to move me along toward where you think I ought to be. Sometimes I'm despairing. Come in here with me. Sometimes I'm optimistic. Come hope with me. Maybe I'm denying the truth. Tell a bald-faced lie with me. Sometimes I'm wallowing. Get in there with me and get dirty, too. I don't need a scheduler. I need not to be alone where I am.

Do The Next Thing. Don't try to figure out how I'll get to radiation every day if I'm sick. Maybe I won't get sick and you'll have made plans that didn't need to be made. Don't talk to me about hospice until I talk about it. Don't talk to me about buying a wig until I want to go buy one. Don't talk to me about nausea until I tell you I'm going to throw up. Don't ask me if I have a will until I say I'm seeing a lawyer. What am I having for dinner tonight? Bake me a casserole. A precious friend who knows cancer brought me a whole meal right out of a dietary book about cancer. It was wonderful and it didn't make me sick from the smell of rich food. Another friend called and asked if I'd read a certain book she liked. I said no. She said, "I'll be right over with it." Then she drove to the bookstore, bought it, and dropped it off. Another friend, dealing with her own illness (not cancer) brought me a potted plant for the front porch. She came by twice without telling me and changed the plants with the seasons.

Do The Little Thing. Can't see yourself holding my head while I throw up? Come load my dishwasher. Don't have the time to spend the day with me while I'm crying? Leave me a note and a dozen cookies. Can't bear the sight of me because I look green and I'm bald? I don't blame you. Send me a new scarf. A nightshirt. A pair of sweats. Write me a letter. (I miss you.)

Don't Tell Me Who Died. I know enough people who are dying. I'm afraid I might be one of them. Don't talk to me about people who are dying or have died of cancer when I don't even know them.

Do Tell Me Who's Living Despite The Odds. I want to hear all the stories about miracles. My favorites are about people who had terrible cancers twenty years ago when we knew next to nothing and are still living despite dire predictions. (I love it that cancer doesn't bat a thousand.) Tell me about people who were fractions of an inch from death and rallied and the treatments worked. Tell me especially about people who have had it worse than me and now it's all a dim memory for them. Nothing beats success. Don't tell me I look just like your Aunt Eula Mae a week before she died.

Don't Ask Me How I Got It. I know what you want—you want to do a checklist of stuff we don't have in common so you'll know where you stand. If my mother had cancer, or I smoke, or I'm fat, or I didn't have checkups, or I didn't have my children until I was thirty, you'll feel better. I won't. I'll feel like you blame me for my cancer.

Don't Tell Me To Quit Reading About It. I have an obsession about cancer now. I want to know everything. Yes, sometimes I read too much and unnecessarily scare myself. It's a way of trying to get control. You think you wouldn't want to know so much. I hope you never find out how much you want to know. And if I don't want to know anything, don't feed me information you think I should have. I'm doing what I have to. If you ever get cancer, I'll try to let you do it your way.

Help Me Laugh. It's a roller coaster. Don't think we have to be serious all the time. One friend called and said, "I just called because I need to be cheered up." "You mean, cheer *me* up," I said. "Heck no," she told me. "I figure after I talk to you I'll feel like Cinderella by comparison." We laughed our heads off. The truth feels great.

Don't Tell Me How Great I'm Doing. I am barely holding on. If my grip slips, have I failed you? Maybe I'm doing great because I'm having an easier time of it than most people. What if it gets worse and I'm a big baby? What will you tell me then? Don't tell me how much you admire me. I have no idea what you're talking about but I suspect it's because I haven't needed you much yet. When a baby is easy to please, doesn't cry much, sleeps through the night, and sticks to a schedule, we say, "What a good baby!" The ones who aren't good babies are the ones who are so much trouble. They can't help it. Neither can I.

Forgive Me Everything. I have no idea what I'm doing. I can't remember my own birthday, much less yours. Sometimes I'll want to talk your head off and the next time you call, I'll cut you off. I don't mean to. I'll correct you, contradict you, irritate you, ignore you, forget to thank you, and make you uncomfortable. Please, please forgive me. I hope to be myself again one day. This is not my finest hour.

And whatever you do, whether it helps or hurts, I'll forgive *you*. Just don't leave me alone in this.

CHAPTER ONE

Headlong Into The Fray

BOLT OUT OF THE BLUE
by Helen Rash

A woman who was a colleague of mine once said, "I never planned to have a career, but I woke up one day and I was having one."

Like many women of my generation, I didn't start out with the idea that I would be earning a living and paying my own bills. It just happened. When I was in high school I didn't really have any role models for what I would later encounter. Among my friends' parents and others in my community I knew teachers, nurses, and women who worked in stores. Most women of that era were married and stayed at home while their husbands worked. As I grew up, I assumed I would follow suit.

After I went to work for the government as a human resources manager, most of my decisions about which job to take next were very unstructured and based on chance. As it turned out, they were good decisions. During the first twenty years of my career I had a series of intelligent, compassionate supervisors and a variety of interesting assignments. In my mid-forties I began finding myself in situations where I had more work than I could handle in a regular 40-hour week, or I had to deal with supervisors whose styles were very different from mine. In spite of these factors, my salary grew, and I continued to receive good recommendations, even from those very supervisors. I gradually arrived at a level which was considered to be very successful in my chosen field.

But I was becoming "angry" about "Work." This did not relate to a particular person but more to what I thought Work had taken from me. I would find myself saying something which turned out to be rather prophetic: "The government has gotten their pound of flesh from me, and they can't have any more." At the very moment when I was successful and felt very welcome by the management of my organization, most of whom were men, I began to see that I had been seduced into a high-adrenaline type of worklife which was going to harm me if I didn't stop it.

Because I was single and had no one dependent on me, I had the luxury of looking for a job which might be less stressful, even if I had to take a cut in pay. In October of 1989 I found such a job and took a $5,000 reduction in salary and a lower government rank in the hopes that I could regain some additional time for my personal life. The day that I realized how much I would miss my friends and colleagues at my old Defense job, I sat in the parking garage of a shopping center and leaned against the steering wheel, sobbing. As I went through the toll booth, the attendant saw my swollen face and asked if I was all right. I gestured with my hand and smiled rather weakly so she'd know not to worry.

I decided that during the last week at my old job I should take the time for a thorough physical, something I'd been doing annually my whole adult life. I had always been in virtually perfect health and so went in with no great concerns. During the exam my doctor ran his hand lightly across the skin of my right breast at about the "two o'clock" position...at the top and toward the center of my chest. He said, "I feel something there." He sent me downstairs to the radiology clinic for a mammogram. (I had had only one mammogram, in 1984, when I had a cyst in my left breast. At that time I had been terrified, but I was referred to a wonderful surgeon who was able to aspirate the fluid with a needle.)

The annual physical took place on a Monday, and by Wednesday the results of the mammogram were ready. When the call came from my doctor, I was at home sitting in front of my stereo, recording some music on tapes. He told me that I needed to see a surgeon as soon as possible and that I should drop by his office to pick up the films so I could carry them with me. After I hung up I got out a bottle of wine and, sitting cross-legged on the floor, I sobbed and drank the wine until it made me sick. I don't normally drink much, but I was trying to dull the pain of the news I'd just received. I had a reaction which I now know is typical of women who take good care of themselves...don't smoke, don't eat or drink to excess. I kept saying, "Why me? I've tried so hard to do the right thing. I even changed jobs to make sure I'd be O.K." At this point all I knew was that there was some evidence of a problem in the mammogram, but the possibilities for disaster reeled out in front of me in long dark lines.

I called several friends but decided not to tell my family about this until I knew what was really happening. My friend Diane offered to go with me to see my surgeon the next Monday. I planned to report to my new job that day and then take the afternoon off, go pick her up, get the mammogram films, and then go on to the surgeon.

The next two days I moved along steadily through work and all the farewells to people, operating on almost no sleep and consuming a great deal of coffee and colas. I told only a few close friends in the office about my test results, since I didn't want to spend my remaining time explaining anything this personal over and over. Besides, I had decided to do something incredibly romantic in the middle of this very difficult time.

The man who was head of the organization where I was working that fall of 1989 was a tall, intellectual military officer who had recently gone through a divorce. Many people viewed him as being overly serious and rather severe, but I had had a chance to talk with him alone on several occasions and knew that he was actually very kind and had a sense of humor. I had also seen a very human side to this man. One day I was wearing a royal blue silk dress with large green dots on it, and he came into my office and said, "That's a wonderful dress!" He did this in a very courteous and nonsexual way, and I enjoyed the compliment. Because he was my second-level supervisor, I couldn't be flirtatious with him or in any way pursue my interest in getting to know him better. However, when I found out I was leaving, I decided to do something which, for me, was rather brazen.

I bought a nice blank greeting card with an oriental painting on the outside and wrote a note to him, saying that I'd certainly enjoyed working for him, and that if he ever wanted to go to the movies or to dinner, I would enjoy that. I enclosed one of my personal calling cards so that he would have my home address and phone number.

I didn't want him to have the note until my last day in the office, because I was feeling a bit awkward about how he would react. I felt that if he received it when I wasn't his employee anymore, and he wasn't interested, then I would be saved the embarrassment of facing him. And so, on that final Friday when I was stoked up with nerve and caffeine, I gave the card to my secretary and asked her to put it into his mail. That was about 7:00 in the morning. About 8:15 I looked up and out the door of my office and saw him moving straight toward my desk, taking his usual long strides, with a wide grin on his face. I sensed immediately that he'd gotten the note and was going to acknowledge it in person. Oh dear!

He came in without hesitation and said, "That was a really nice thing to do." Then he added that he probably would call me some time. He handled the situation very well and when he turned to leave, I felt that what I'd done was all right. It was a bright spot in an otherwise very bad week. It also gave me some sense that life might hold something other than the fear which I was feeling at that moment.

THOSE LITTLE VOICES INSIDE YOUR HEAD
by Judy Klevins

Watching TV in bed and coughing with a three-week cold, I warmed my hands in my armpits. I felt something on my right breast. It itched a bit, so I scratched it and thought I had a hive, or a mosquito bite that would go away in an hour. It didn't. I convinced myself it would go away by Monday.

The vocal director of the musical had encouraged me to take time off for my cold so I would be in good shape for the two weeks before opening night, so I called her. She and the assistant director and stage manager agreed to take over Monday's killer first-rehearsal-without-script-or-cues. It was the first rehearsal I had missed in over twenty-five years of directing.

Monday morning

A schizophrenic dialogue began before I opened my eyes.

A: *Better check your breast out.*

B: *Why do that now, of all times; you can't deal with that now!*

A: *If you don't do it now, you'll deal with it subconsciously anyway.*

B: *Just ignore it: maybe it will go away! Besides, you were just at the doctor's yesterday; they'll think you're stupid...you're just looking for attention, for an excuse not to do your work. Yeah, you're just letting your imagination run away with you again...nothing is wrong.*

A: *Shut up...we're calling the doctor.*

Friday afternoon

After my physical and preliminary aspiration, a biopsy was ordered. For a lump all doctors said looked "O.K.," a lot of appointments were being made.

I went to the library to find out more about cancer. Some of the books were medical tomes. Many books had contradictory advice and information. Some showed how wonderful you could look bald with snazzy stars on your pate. One book on chemotherapy made me sick to my stomach. How could I ever handle the reality? I could only read *Up Front. Sex and the Post-Mastectomy Woman,* because I thought I would never have sex again, so I couldn't identify with these people with cancer.

Monday afternoon

I remember the operating room, the friendly staff and being transferred from the gurney to a really narrow table. I asked what they did with fat patients. I was being strapped in…someone said "Judy, Judy, wake up." I thought I was late for school. Then someone told me the lump was malignant…my friend and I started to cry. I don't remember that night.

SUICIDE IS OPTIONAL
by Katherine Traynham

I would never, never take my own life. It is an act of despicable cowardice. It is probably immoral. It is a vindictive, vengeful act of malice towards those who love you. That's how I felt. I knew this part of me was immutable. The way you know you're not the kind of mother who would ever burn her child with cigarettes.

But cancer introduces you to the person you really are—not the one you've invented. I hear people say, "The God I believe in would never do that. The God I believe in is like this...," and then they explain. I always wondered, "What if the God you believe in isn't the God who really is?" And now I know the person I believed I was had little resemblance to the person I really am.

Here is the person I really am: Suicide was my second thought. My first thought was: Thank God it's not my husband or children. I held my mother's hand while she died of cancer. I fed drops of juice to a dear friend who died of cancer. I know what it is to be the person who isn't dying and it nearly killed me anyway. If you're going to be nearly killed, you might as well be the one dying.

Then, the next thought: I will take myself out before it nearly kills them.

Sometimes, because I am thoughtless and like to go for the laugh, and because an Irish temper is not the most attractive ethnic feature in my family, I have heard something said that is outrageous, and I have literally thought, "Who said *that?*" in the moment before I realized it had come out of *my* mouth.

This was like that. I thought, "I will take myself out before it nearly kills them, and I know exactly how I will do it." And I thought, "Who is that, thinking of suicide in my head?"

How can you know how you will kill yourself if you've never thought of it before? There was chaos in my head. The doctor was talking to me, comforting my tears. The nurse was in and out. My husband was stricken, looking at me and the doctor as if we had just dropped in out of the sky. I heard and perceived all that was going on, and although sedated from surgery, I was recording it all. Meanwhile, my brain had quickly flipped to a file I didn't know I'd stored. The title was, "Instructions on How to Kill Myself, If the Need Ever Arises."

When had I worked on that project? How was it completed without my knowledge? Where was it stored, completely unfiltered from what I knew to be my faith, my belief system? How did it escape my heart-searchings? Where was the cabinet in which it had hidden, and what the hell else was in there that I don't know about?

Do philosophers still believe "to know oneself" is the greatest work of life? And how exactly do they propose that we do that, when we have no idea what little plans have been cooked up while we are not aware?

I was not thinking of suicide because I was in terrible pain. I wasn't, and wasn't about to be. I wasn't thinking of suicide because I had become a shell of myself, after a thousand humiliating instances of dependence as my dignity shredded itself and sloughed away. I was not contemplating killing myself because I had become a hopeless burden to those who loved me and the seeing it in their eyes was much worse than dying and not ever seeing their eyes again.

I was not about to die any time soon. I might even live a long, long time. There was every reason to think, in that moment, that I would die of something else besides cancer, and certainly something besides this cancer. I had to literally "read the notes" on this hidden file to find out what my reasons were. Here's what was there: 1. *I do not want my husband and children to see what I saw with my mother, and hers was easy compared to what I've heard from others. 2. I do not want them to spend a fortune caring for me if this drags out and be impoverished if I only die anyway. 3. I do not want my husband to see me become something he takes care of that used to be a lover but will never be again. 4. I do not want to say good-bye to them or to life, slowly, a million times, in tiny little good-byes. ("The coward dies a thousand deaths, etc.") And finally, the "note" that was attached that makes me so ashamed:*

5. This will be a dramatic ending. I won't be the wife who faded away from cancer, leaving memories that make them cringe. It will be a fast, big-bang kind of thing. In that way, I'll have a better chance of still being the love of my husband's life, even if he has twenty or thirty years with some other woman.

This cancer is a terrible thing. It does what it does, it goes where it goes, it kills what it will. That's not the worst of it. The worst of it is you find out. You find out who you are. What you really think. Where the dark places are. Tell yourself what you want about what you believe and what you'd do. Just don't swear on a Bible until it happens and you go through all the files in .0006 of a second to see what comes up.

I don't want this to be me. I even have hope that I will have time to change who I am before a moment comes that requires a real decision. But for now, this is who I am. I have to admit that because I don't tell anybody the "how" that's in the file. They might figure out a way to keep me from doing it someday. I tell them everything except that. Because that's really who I am. Someone who might just kill herself rather than face it the way it comes.

GET A SECOND OPINION
by Daena Kluegel

Hospitals are not warm and welcoming places, however they are decorated. They can dress all the staff in pretty print or pastel outfits but a hospital is still a place usually entered with some foreboding. I had come on a dreary cold and gray January morning for a biopsy. We grimly approached the hospital entrance and, once inside, we were surrounded by bustle and bright lights. I was hungry, thirsty and, in spite of the Valium, very uneasy. The staff bustled around preparing for the "procedure," as they called it. Ken and I answered questions and filled out yet more insurance information forms. I wondered, "Where is the surgeon?" and "Where is the order for Valium, preoperatively?" The staff was not unfriendly, just efficient and lacking in time for human contact. Modern healing, as housed in a modern hospital and issued by a trained modern staff, bears no resemblance to the kindly, unselfish, and motivated characters seen on *St. Elsewhere* and *E.R.* On those shows, I'm sure I've never seen anyone asking patients insurance related questions.

What was I doing here? I remembered again the panic which tightened my gut when I found The Lump. It was Martin Luther King, Jr. Day. I crawled into bed after a busy day. I started my routine Breast Self-Exam. My thoughts drifted as I felt my own familiar flesh and tissue. As I moved my fingers around the right breast, they encountered a hard, round area under the skin near the nipple. I stopped, now I was fully awake, adrenaline pumping. I began again. Yes, there it was. I tried to calmly check if there was a similar something in the same position on the left breast. Was there anything there? Could I have mistaken something normal? *No*, that was indeed a false hope. I kept touching it.

Ethel's face came back to me. My kindly friend who had been my aide in the classroom for thirteen years had died two years earlier of breast cancer. Ethel was my only contact with a "victim." "Well, tomorrow, I'll call my doctor," I thought as I tried to calm down, stop squirming, and sleep.

So, I went to my gynecologist. She reassured me but I persisted and finally she sent me for a mammogram that day. The lump was never found on the mammogram, but it was located by sonogram. "No risk factors, but it is hard, so it will have to be biopsied. Don't worry, most lumps are benign." "It's regular in shape, so don't worry." "It's in the wrong breast and wrong quadrant, so don't worry." I wanted to believe, but I was worried. Had I done something to deserve this? What had my glasses of wine and lunches of cheese and paté done to my breasts?

"He's here, and here is your Valium; we'll be using a local when we get to the O.R." I was accompanied to the doors of a cold, white room where I sat on the table. They explained everything as they began. They introduced me to the "team." One nurse told me that she would stay in close contact with me, holding my hand if I liked. She said she'd had the same procedure and knew how difficult and frightening it was. She would, she said, "Be there for you," in a pleasant voice, smiling and sincere. I was relieved and grateful for her presence. They covered my head with a towel so I couldn't see what they were doing. I was grateful, as I was busy trying to distance myself from the whole procedure by making mental lists, (an old defense mechanism for me in times of difficulty).

The surgeon was explaining things to another younger doctor as he went. The tones were routine and the speech subdued. Then I heard, "My God! It's deeper than I thought. Look, there's the fascia!" There was a sudden, ominous silence.

My special nurse hastily interrupted, "Oh, it's time for my lunch break. I have to go." She dropped my hand and left, promising to send someone to replace her.

The surgeon left with the tissue specimen shortly thereafter and the younger physician stitched up my incision. As I was wheeled to Recovery, the surgeon passed me in the corridor. One look at his face told me all I needed to know. He looked upset, red-faced, strangely defeated from his bushy black hair and bristly eyebrows to his limp hands. He mumbled something about meeting us in Recovery. I sat dumbly, mute in my agonizing terror, while the smells of alcohol and disinfectant and the sounds of staff busily putting away instruments in preparation for the next procedure flooded my senses and added to my fear.

My husband Ken was waiting in the cubicle. The surgeon entered. "I'm sorry; it is bad news; it is malignant," he blurted out and left. I glanced at Ken. How pale he'd become...then Ken slid against the wall and fainted. I thought I'd hyperventilate, it was so hard to breathe. I gasped for air frantically as the bands of fear tightened around my lungs while my heartbeat pulsed the blood in my temples. I was feeling like a squashed bug, but I did notice Ken and asked them to help him.

After Ken was revived, we had the sense to ask for a second opinion on the frozen tissue sample. The nurse told us to call for an appointment with the surgeon. I got dressed and the two lost souls wandered off in despair.

At least no one said, "Have a nice day."

We found out about second opinions. We even found out about third and fourth opinions. Then our network of friends went into action and we found a more humane man for our surgeon and a teaching hospital for my mastectomy. Those nurses were really caring and kind. When I sensed a lack of rapport with one team of oncologists, we found a much better and nicer man who treated me with respect and credited my intellect. We had to learn to seek out and question alternatives when we were least able to do so. We learned quickly and were very aware of the atmosphere in the offices and the staff in them. This helped us select the reconstructive surgeon to join our team. Never again did I let anyone show me a callous or inhumane attitude. Once, I was kept waiting a very long time so I marched out into the office in my tissue paper examining gown and asked loudly how long I could expect to wait to see the doctor. When the doctor came in rather hurriedly, he was very apologetic and the nurse was never seen again.

I returned to the gynecologist. She questioned my change in surgeons and hospitals and even why I'd had chemotherapy. "You should not have done that; now you are in premature menopause and your vagina will atrophy." I drove home in tears, but I calmed down and had all my records sent to a new gynecologist.

Moral: Don't let the Medical Establishment become your god and make your decisions for you. Confront, question, seek alternatives, and listen to your own best judgment. I hope this message comes clearly through my story. You may never meet such uncaring, callous medical personnel (and I sincerely hope you will not). But you do not have to remain in this situation. Women have been brought up not to question, to follow and be "good." You do have choices in your medical treatment, your life and death. One woman brought me to my senses in the midst of despair when she practically shook me and said, "Get a second opinion and get to a teaching hospital!" She made all the difference in my treatment.

FEAR (0-8 MONTHS)
by Katherine Traynham

In the middle of my life, or what I thought would be,
was this train wreck. A terrifying conflagration.

A massacre, complete with blood and guts and screaming.

One day, I was just walking along in my life—piddling.
Piddling with the dishes, the kids, the friends, the lists of things,
the needlework, the dusting.
And then the next, I was exploded. In pieces, and torn.
In terrible need of a trauma team, only no one noticed.
For the explosion was in my head, and the crash
Only my soul colliding with a single word:
Cancer.

(How can such a common thing make such terror?)
No one attacked me on the street. I was not raped by a stranger
but a familiar.
No one burned my house or stole my babies. There are worse
terrors in the night—
And yet.

And yet, this black Thing came and sat beside me.
He was old and dark and empty, and I knew if I didn't WATCH IT,
he could make me stop breathing.
I wanted him away, yet the important thing became to
just keep breathing.
Despite him. To keep thinking. To keep hearing. To keep living.
To keep me.
And the waves of fear that he was
Kept washing over me.

I felt betrayed all over again. By every I love you that wasn't
with me still.
By every kiss and promise.

By every part of this mad system that says,
"We know. You can trust us." And we trust and we are still attacked.
They say, "A dis-ease. Your heredity. Your habits. Did you follow the rules? Did you become a woman too early? Did you time your babies wrong? Have the wrong aunt? Mother? Grandmother? No matter. We can do so much."
(And then you must do more.)
You must pray and exercise and eat certain foods and meditate and laugh and stay away from hard things that make you cry and you must do all that NEVER WAVERING.
And take your vitamins.

And then I will live? I say.
Maybe.
Maybe not.
And now, after weeks and weeks of willing it and praying it,
The black Thing has moved to the street, not sitting beside me anymore.
But it's not far.
I will him to the horizon. I practice levitating him into the sea.

My safest place is gone—that mother who was always calm.
That refuge that loved me even if I had eaten wrong, not exercised, not meditated.
She who let me be bad and loved me anyway is now in the truly safe place
(and I am glad). I don't want her to see me now. I want her for me and yet I know she was powerless against these Things. She would never bow to them, but arrayed against me
They would terrorize her.

So. I take my vitamins. I don't tell anyone that sometimes, once in awhile, I still smoke. Because they will frown and shake their heads and give up on me.
They can't do the hard things themselves. The things I have done.

But they will shake their heads sadly and give up on me if I cannot do the next hard thing they assign.

So. I am a trooper. A good scout. I go to where they put the poison in my veins. The male doctors get mad if we call it poison. It poisons the cancer, I tell them. They don't hear the difference.

(They are reading the same books I do about positive attitude.) I go to where they burn my chest with radiation. They don't want me to call it burning. I tell them they are burning away the bad flesh.

They don't hear the difference. They want me to endorse what they have to do to me.

What I want them to do to me.

I start to think that men, especially in medicine, have a hearing problem.

I promised not to count up again, how many times I have not been heard by men.

To count up the kisses. The ones who went away. The ones who went away mad.

And now, these. Who want me to give my body a whole new way and not be angry if it doesn't work.

Too much to ask, don't you think?

Virginity was easy to give away, compared to this.

And when I'm sick, and furious, and counting betrayals,

And waiting for the next ones, and shaking and still trying to shove the black Thing out to the horizon now and get him far enough away

He's there. The anti-betrayer. The anti-deserter. The anti-doctor.

He's been here all along, and because I don't trust many of his kind I flat-out forgot.

I haven't told him I'm afraid I will die no matter what we do.

He knows. And after several months, he tells me he knows. In an oblique way.

As if it were about someone else. That he knows women must

lie there in the night and wonder if it will kill them, sooner or later. Every night.

And it is more wondrous because I didn't tell him.

He knew, because he has slept beside me for ten years. He has watched my face.

He is listening with his heart.

I have tried not to look into his face so much because the pain and fear were tortuous at first.

I always wanted to make him smile—not that easy—or laugh outright—nearly impossible—and never be the cause of this thing in his face.

And yet.

And yet he says it is the most important thing that ever happened to us. (It isn't—the children or God or WE are, but not this.)

But I love it that he thinks it is. That he thinks it has happened to us, not just to me.

Like a grand warrior from the Bible, he stands there in the gap, between us and disaster.

He stands in the gap when I am afraid to cross over. He stands, a bridge between me and our future.

He doesn't seem to care about scars and burnings. He doesn't seem to care that I look nothing like myself. He doesn't seem to notice that

I am not myself and can't be again.

He gets angry when I talk about what it costs. He will not talk about what if it comes back.

I love him for that too, more than he can know.

I haven't told him everything. I never will.

But I don't need my mother anymore. He is doing a better job than she could have.

He has the heart for it. And the courage.

And I don't tell him what I first told God when they said, "Cancer."

I told Him, "Thank you that it's me and not him or the children."

I don't speak it out loud anymore.

I am getting superstitious about the Thing. It's out on the ocean somewhere.

I don't ever want it so close again. It won't ever surprise me like that again.

It was just the train wreck. In the middle of my life. That's what surprised me.

So, I tell God in my mind, in the voice He always hears.

Thank you! A million times. My children are well. My husband stands in the gap.

Let what comes come.

I will be busy living.

CHAPTER TWO

Facing It—Alone, Together
Alone With Someone

PRUNING
by Helen Rash

I began my new job on October 30, 1989, and went to see the surgeon that afternoon. This was the man who'd aspirated the cyst in my left breast in 1984, and I liked him very much. He was quite bright and skilled and yet extremely tender-hearted. I left work in Arlington, drove up into D.C. to pick up Diane, and the two of us went out to Maryland to my oncologist's to get the mammogram films. We went from there to the surgeon's office where he studied the file and talked to me about the need for a biopsy. It was scheduled for November 16.

In my diary on October 31, I wrote only this: "Yesterday I went to see the surgeon. On November 16, I will have the lump removed." The next day I wrote: "I slept well last night until 3:00. Then I cried. Then an image came into my head. It had to do with autumn and the fact that trees lose their leaves. But, the trees are still whole through the winter, and they blossom again after resting. My acupuncturist has often talked about the fall season, how it's a time to let go, but it's also a beginning, a harvest." I had been to see him a few days earlier, and he had said perhaps this "thing" in my breast needed to come out, and then I could put all the recent pains and problems behind me.

During the next two weeks I was very anxious, not knowing what the surgery would be like or whether the spot on the mammogram would, in fact, turn out to be a malignancy. I had trouble sleeping, and work was difficult because it was new and I had only half the employees I was supposed to have. I was interviewing candidates, but in the meantime I was short of help.

Diane drove me to the biopsy, which was a fast and painless procedure done under general anesthesia. I was sitting in the recovery area when my surgeon came to see me with the results of the biopsy. It was cancer, but very small. He said I should see him the next day, which was a Friday. That Thursday night I spent with my friends Robert and Michelle and their two young daughters. From their house I called my brother to let him know the results. I wanted him to be able to go and see my mother before she learned what had happened. When I knew that he had gotten to her apartment, I called to talk with her.

The next day Michelle and my little redheaded goddaughter Emily and I snuggled up in bed together with some rented videos. Emily had a "sore throat" which I suspect was really an excuse to stay home from school and be with us. Late in the afternoon Michelle went with me to see the surgeon. He'd read the official pathologist's report by that time, and he said there were many options; but he recommended a lumpectomy followed by radiation. I cried, and he hugged me.

When I went out to the reception area, Michelle was talking with one of the patients, an attractive woman who looked to be in her forties. She introduced herself. My doctor asked her if she would be willing to show me her breasts, because two years earlier she'd had a lumpectomy. He took us back into his office, gave us cold drinks, and left us with Marcia. When she opened her sweater, what I saw was a woman with normal breasts. There was a slight scar from the surgery, but other than that, there was no evidence that anything had happened. This was a tremendous turning point for me, knowing that I could be whole again. I was further encouraged when my surgeon said we'd caught the cancer early.

I began to feel more relaxed, because suddenly I had a sense of what might happen. Before this I could only picture my chest with one full, well-formed breast and a big gaping hole on the other side. I'd had only one acquaintance who'd had a mastectomy, my belly-dancing teacher. She'd had her operation in the early 1970's, when women were asked to sign a release as they went into surgery, giving permission to the surgeons to do whatever they saw fit while operating. This meant that the woman would awaken and look down at her breasts, not knowing whether there would be one or two...a totally barbaric practice which is no longer used.

After the biopsy I developed a severe hematoma, and my breast turned purple and yellow. My doctor had to open the small incision to release the pressure of the blood, a procedure which was very grueling both physically and emotionally. The Saturday after Thanksgiving I was to attend a dinner party at Robert and Michelle's, and that afternoon I took a nap so that I would be ready to go out that night. When I awoke I found that I was bleeding spontaneously from the little slit in my breast. I was terribly upset and called my surgeon immediately. He was out of town, but I was referred to his colleague, who told me that this was a natural thing and actually was good, because it would help drain that area. He told me to put sterile compresses on it and a heating pad. I called Michelle in tears to explain and told her I didn't even have any bandages in the house. She told me to hang on, that they would be right over with the supplies and that I was to come and sleep at their house, even if I didn't feel like being at the party.

And so they held onto me and adopted me and gave me their older daughter's bed, where I rested and ate food brought on a tray by Robert. It was this kind of support that was to see me through a lot of difficult times. The next morning I slipped out of their house quietly, leaving a five-dollar bill on the table for the bandages. They later really let me have it over the five dollars, saying I needed to learn to accept this kind of simple help. I explained that one big issue with my kind of medical problem was that life seemed so out of control, and that trying to be independent and normal was so important…thus the effort to pay my own way. I promised that next time I wouldn't feel compelled to worry about the money.

On Wednesday, November 29, the surgeon removed a small wedge from my breast and some of the lymph nodes under my right arm. My friend Gretchen went with me. I immediately felt very good, both physically and emotionally. I was willing to show my bosom to almost anyone who'd look, so pleased was I to have two very normal, perky breasts. There were lots of cards, company, and flowers.

Pattie, who lived just around the corner from the hospital, came to take me home on Saturday; and we dropped by Baskin-Robbins for one of our favorite things: hot fudge sundaes. The next day Diane took me to the grocery store to make sure I had food in the house. That night my oncologist called, and when I heard his voice I knew that there had to be something wrong or he wouldn't have called me at that time. He said they had found cancer in some of the lymph nodes, and that we needed to talk. I cried myself to sleep.

Monday I took a day off from work and got a crown put on one of my teeth. I'd broken the tooth while eating a grape my last day in the hospital. When this had happened, I'd just sat on the bed, smiling and shaking my head. It seemed a rather minor aggravation in the middle of all the other problems. That night my former boss, with whom I'd flirted as I left the old job, called me, and we had a nice talk. He said he was going out of town, but that he planned to call me soon so we could have dinner. It was just the boost I needed.

In retrospect, I probably should have taken more time to heal, but I felt all right and thought I was ready to return to work. By Wednesday I was very feverish and felt strange. I didn't know at the time that I had developed a severe post-op infection. Since I was to see my surgeon the next day, I didn't bother to call him. On Thursday I went first to the oncologist's office, accompanied by Marcia, the woman I'd met through my surgeon.

CAN YOU COME HERE WHERE I AM?

She had insisted that she go with me, since I was very sure I would be hearing that I needed chemotherapy in addition to radiation, now that we knew I had positive lymph nodes. I appreciated her moral support. Her mother had been a breast-cancer patient of my oncologist, so Marcia was no stranger. We did, in fact, discuss chemotherapy, which we scheduled to start on December 13. The six weeks of radiation would run simultaneously but would not begin until January. Marcia was able to share with me that her mother had gone through chemo without nausea and without losing her hair. Knowing this helped me a great deal.

In the late afternoon I went on to my surgeon's office. He was terribly upset about the infection and immediately called my doctor to postpone the start of the chemo until we could get things cleared up through some powerful antibiotics. The drugs began working immediately, and my spirits lifted a bit.

Since I knew that I would be going out on a date soon, I set aside the next Saturday to be good to myself. I went shopping with Gretchen, who's very skilled at putting clothes and jewelry together. She took me to a very expensive boutique in suburban Virginia, where I tried on piles of gorgeous outfits. This was a very important moment. I was still wearing bandages, but my body looked good, and I spent $1,500 on three outfits. To this day I don't regret a penny of it. I had my hair done that day and had dinner with friends. I was starting to feel "normal."

On the day I was to have begun chemotherapy, I instead had a very pleasant dinner date with the tall, nice officer from work. I wore one of my new dresses and felt very good about the evening. As I had expected, he was a gentleman and fun to talk to. We spent our time discussing places we had visited in Europe and the Orient. I didn't need or want a man to come on to me sexually, since I was just getting over the surgery and still dealing with the incision. It was enough to feel slightly glamorous and to do things other women were doing. In my diary I wrote: "My spirits are great—and I'm physically strong. I feel like my life is opening up in front of me!"

ALONE
by Katherine Traynham

Don't be alone
the doctor said
For awhile
keep people nearby
Don't be alone
with just yourself
until you feel better

But I couldn't wait
to get them out
Away from the house
and from my rooms
Where I could pace
and cry and mourn
and play the piano

And I would wail
and wring my hands
And flutter though
family knickknacks
Evoking names and
memories of those
Gone on ahead

I'd play old songs
and weep for them
And conjure up
the newly dead
And wrap myself
in tragedy
For heartbreak's sake

Eventually, I got to where
I bored myself

Can You Come Here Where I Am?

With vacantness
and even my
Mortality
lost its infinite
fascination

It came to pass
that I ran out
Of melodrama
starring me
And somewhere near
the denouement
I left the theater

Left alone
even I will start to
Yawn eventually
and no one holds
The center stage
who stars, directs
and rents a box

Don't be alone
and watch the same
Production of your misery
unless you also
Have the nerve to
take the critic's chair
near the exit

It should have closed
that first night
But the backer hadn't
any sense
And so it dragged
through several acts
And too few rewrites

These one-woman shows
(don't be alone)
Are bigger than life
(don't be alone)
But now, ensemble roles
are what I seek
And I feel better.

FEED YOUR HEAD
by Katherine Traynham

Some of us remember the "natural childbirth" movement. This is the one where we trudged off every week for a couple of months to some place where a "trainer" would teach us how to breathe so we would be able to do twenty-six hours of back labor without poisoning our child-to-be with so much as a Tylenol. We'd be gently massaged by our husbands. We'd crunch ice chips. We'd concentrate on the poster of some hunk in "Playgirl" or a pastoral scene from a travel magazine. We wouldn't need an episiotomy, much less anesthesia. We'd just gently dilate until our precious slipped sweetly into the hands of the doctor, after a few muted grunts and lots of counting from our husband, the coach.

It was a great theory. It even worked for a lot of women. We were rebelling against the drug generation, maybe? Some of us smoked street dope we got from strangers but once we got pregnant considered Demerol a definite toxin. Or maybe it was about the time the news magazines reported the over-medication of all our grandparents in nursing homes, or the plight of the American housewife hooked on diet pills and Valium, in between 5:00 p.m. highballs.

At any rate, we decided it was best not to dull the pain—to get right in there with it and feel whatever you have to feel and work through it. To experience all of life, even its momentary miseries. We would be pure. We would be purged. We would not scream.

My sister said, "TAKE THE EPIDURAL."

Since then, there have been a lot of swell drugs developed. I, of course, being the purist who believes you really can only take one ibuprofen at a time, no matter how bad your head hurts, and you really do have to wait exactly eight hours from one dose of Nyquil to the next, felt like a wimp when my husband said to the doctor, "Can you give her something?"

It was three weeks since my diagnosis and I was shattered. Weepy. Terrorized. Oh, I thought I was handling it okay. I thought everybody who had cancer probably read 6,000 pages a day of medical journals. I made my husband go to a medical school bookstore at a nearby university and buy me what the med students were reading about cancer and chemotherapy. I bought a textbook on lumpectomy surgery. I found a place that would send me summaries on the companies that made the chemotherapy chemicals. And this was only week three. Wait till we get to the radiation part and the machines and how they're calibrated.

"Can you give her something?" my husband wanted to know, with a tinge of desperation in his voice. And the doctor agreed an anti-anxiety drug was in order.

In four days, I began to feel that the world wasn't coming to an end. Or at least might not. That weekend, anyway.

I took it for six weeks. It gave me my mental balance back. But I felt like a wimp. A baby. A big, silly, middle-aged case of nerves. Nobody gave my mother's best friend drugs twenty-five years ago when she got cancer.

Oh, yes they did, I found out later. Valium.

Well, women have been dealing with cancer for centuries, and they all managed without drugs.

Yes, and without anesthesia, or antiseptic soap during births and surgeries, and were carted off to loony bins for postpartum depression and...well, you get the drift.

Young women today still do the childbirth classes. But they also sign the form in advance for the epidural. They don't feel pain relief is a character flaw. They don't make decisions on breast feeding based on high moral principles, but on their preference. They don't ask each other, "How long do you plan to nurse?" in an accusatory tone. In fact, I used the term "natural" childbirth not long ago and one of them corrected me—"All childbirth is natural," she smiled. Well, yes. I mean, what would be "unnatural childbirth?" No, don't tell me.

The point is, if you need medication, take it. Ask for it. Some women don't need it. Some women do. Some of it's for physical pain. Some of it will help the other kind. Thank God it's there if you need it. There should be no guilt in doing whatever you have to, to get through this.

WHAT SHE HEARD, WHAT I SAID
by Katherine Traynham

She doesn't remember it the way I do. We'd sent her to her grandparents' house to look at a college and take the tour. The surgery, supposedly no big deal, just a benign lump or cyst, or whatever, would be while she was gone. She'd be home the next day.

But it was no big deal. And I had reassured her everything would be fine. It was the first time I'd ever lied to her. Every other time in her life, when I'd say, "Everything will turn out okay," it had. This time, I'd been wrong.

We planned it carefully, my husband and I. He believes the worst thing you can do is not tell them, or act as if you don't want to tell them something. He remembers, as a child, believing the absolute worst, when the truth—while scary—wouldn't have been as bad as what he'd imagined.

We went to the airport to pick her up. "How was it? Did you like it? Did you have fun? Did you call Shawn?"

"How was your surgery?"

"Difficult," I said. And then we got her luggage.

Chat, chat, chat, in the car. Then, "So, everything was okay? The lump was nothing?"

Not nothing. And we told her. And she was upset but didn't seem distraught. We answered her questions. She had only a few. And when she got home, she went to her room and cried. My husband went in to talk to her. He told her we would do everything we could to deal with it. That her life, no matter what happened to me, would still be guided by my love for her, and his. Her plans weren't threatened. It would be a hard year, but she didn't need to panic. I was not going to die anytime soon.

That's the only part she remembers. When she described it to someone else weeks later, she says she was so shocked she went into a trance. She doesn't remember it being "later" that we talked. She thinks she got off the plane and we said, "Hello. It's cancer," or something like that. She remembers that she thought that meant I was going to die right away. She thought of a friend whose mother has battled cancer for years. She always felt sorry for him. Now she felt sorry for herself.

She thinks it was the next day that my husband came into her room—not a few hours after she got home. She does remember feeling better after he reassured her. She has no memory of how calm we were, or how normal we tried to be. She only remembers the panic.

Is there a good way to do this? Did we miss something? Was there a moment we missed, or is it just too hard to tell a 16-year-old something that might change her life forever, too? Was I the one in a trance? Do I remember it right? I remember telling her right away that my having cancer meant she would need to be vigilant about it as an adult, because it increases her chances some. Did I need to tell her that then, just because it was on my mind?

One of us was not paying attention. Not "in the moment." Not absorbing the exchange we had. I think it might have been me. I think she may remember it "right"—instead of how it really happened. She heard, "Mom's going to die of cancer." I said everything *but* that. But she heard me anyway. I was screaming it in my head. My mouth said, "This can be handled, this is manageable." She didn't hear me. The roar of my fear drowned out everything else.

LOVE STORY
by Katherine Traynham

No doubt most of our friends would be shocked at how I see us. How I think of us. We're neither of us movie stars, and our best days of youth are behind us, for certain. As handsome as my husband is, he's starting to look—not thirty anymore. And I—well, I look like my mother, or someone closely related to her. Motherly. And yet—he and I are lovers, like in old stories, old movies. That's how I see us.

We were already grown-up when we met. Our once-upon-a-time started when we were truly adults—and both already divorced parents. We worked together and whether because of our histories, our personalities, or whatever else, no one who knew us then (with a couple of extreme exceptions) thought we were suited for each other. The unflattering speculation about us often made its way back to our ears.

We never hesitated for a second.

It was New Orleans. After a night with friends, we danced and then he walked me to my car. November in New Orleans is like a delicious spring anywhere else. The river sounds nearby, the lazy stars overhead. And music everywhere. And under a full November moon, in a city that really belongs in Europe, he kissed me in the dark, and I was captured.

It's been nearly fifteen years, and I have a thousand memories of continuing rapture. A million times of a little electrical jolt when he comes in the room, when he turns his head to look at me, when he closes his eyes and laughs out loud, or comes up behind me and puts his head down near mine.

It didn't change when I started turning gray, or got extra lines, or picked up pounds. It hasn't changed through teenage kids or debt or disappointment. Despite daily life and flaws and irritations, I am chagrined at how deeply and helplessly in love with him I still am. It is a secret, vulnerable thing that almost shames me and is my deepest pride.

No one would ever guess we are starring in a love story and that he is my only memory of passion and that soaring youth that makes you reckless. He alone entices me, and he alone has the power to transform me into someone young and beautiful. And despite the hell months of cancer treatment, and the scars that prove it, in every waking moment, I am still a young woman in love with a handsome man, and at any moment, he could take me in his arms under a November moon and capture me with a kiss.

IT'S ABOUT LOVE
by Daena Kluegel

When I married thirty-four years ago, we took vows. These included "for richer or poorer" and "in sickness and in health." Breast cancer was a test which we were given. It was especially hard to pass those two vows, but we did it. It was a very big challenge and one not many men can meet. This daunting task includes helping you feel loved and desirable after surgery and throughout chemotherapy with its nausea and fatigue. He slept in a chair in the hospital room after my surgery and then went home to call all the family and friends. He cleaned and remade our bed when I dumped a pitcher of water on it, on him, and on me, while reaching for a drink with my stiff and weakened arm.

My husband saw how lethargic and depressed I had become following surgery. He said, "Go get the car keys."

"But I don't want to go for a ride," I whined.

"No," he said. "You're driving." It was pretty difficult with my arm still stiff from the node dissection, but I did drive with our standard shift car, and afterward I felt more normal and empowered. He saw my need and found a way for me to overcome it.

One dark February day while I was still striving to resume normal activities like washing my own hair and buttoning a blouse in back, he whisked me out of my despair by taking me for a tour to the greenest of green environments in the winter, the Botanical Gardens. What a difference that made in my outlook.

He never averted his eyes when faced with my surgically scarred body, and he continued to physically assure me of my desirability from the first night I returned from the hospital after surgery. What a relief that was. I have never doubted since then that our attraction was still strong and healthy.

Infinitely kind and with limitless patience, he listened long and hard. Sometimes he made suggestions, sometimes he cried with me, and sometimes he just held and comforted me. He offered me empathy, not sympathy. He was steadfast in his verbal statements about his belief in my ability to win the battle and come through it healthy, and he was willing to help me do that. He cleaned the house and cooked the meals. I expected him to break out in hives because he'd washed so many dishes as a kid, he'd declared after our wedding that he'd never wash another dish. He distracted me and entertained me with humor and great sensitivity.

He could also be hard-eyed and unblinking in his "Brinkmanship games," dealing with the difficult underlings we encountered in the medical or insurance offices. He exercised his ability to cut through to the important and to follow through the sometimes horrific paperwork of medical and insurance forms, payments and treatments. He was my eyes and also my ears during the medical consults because I was overwhelmed much of the time. He spent infinite hours explaining and helping me weigh factors in those important decisions. Was he impatient, complaining? I never knew it.

Most importantly, he was able to forgive and get us as a couple beyond any past problems and move us forward. He was uncomplaining about the insurance and its headaches. He even ignored the dent in our budget left by financing a new wardrobe in a larger size. He planned and financed those vacations I wanted us to take because of my new priorities. Is he a saint? Not yet! But he's certainly working on it.

My dear, these gifts are more meaningful than any of those you brought me in the blue Tiffany's boxes. My love and appreciation for you and your gifts have increased without measure.

WHERE ARE THE MEN?
by Katherine Traynham

Women make a big fuss about my husband. He's a good-looking guy. Six feet, four inches. Dark brown hair and eyes. Smooth skin, square of jaw, and very, very male. The nurses watch him when he comes in. They say they want to make sure he won't bump his head on the door frame. (Oh, sure. That's it.) Female doctors smile reassuringly more often when they talk to him than when they talk to me. A very masculine male makes females feel more so in his presence, I think.

At first, that's all I thought it was. Then one day, at radiation, while sitting in the waiting room, my husband said, "Where are they?"

"Where are who?"

"The men," he said. "Where are all the men?"

There were women there with mothers who were having radiation. There were mothers there with daughters. There were sisters, neighbors, best friends, and a granddaughter. There were women with the few men who were there to have radiation. It was the same at the place we went for my chemo infusion. The male patients came in with wives or daughters. The women came in—alone, or with a female friend.

"Where are they?" My husband insisted on knowing. He began to look for them, but we didn't find any over the next months. He went with me to most chemo treatments. He went with me to doctors appointments. He went with me to some of my radiation treatments over six weeks. We didn't find any husbands besides him. He was a big attraction not because he was a good-looking man. He was a big attraction because he was the only man accompanying a wife with breast cancer. With any cancer, as far as we could tell from the waiting rooms.

My husband travels. He works twelve hours a day on a slow day, when he's not traveling. He can travel, some years, up to 180 days out of 365. When I got cancer, he told them he wouldn't be traveling unless we agreed and it was a short trip. He arranged to take lots of time off, lots of mornings off, lots of time off on short notice. I almost made a terrible mistake.

Because he travels, because he is a man, because I don't want to be "any trouble," I was making plans to have my best friend do everything he wanted to do. Because even if he wanted to do it, I didn't see how he could. With work. With travel. With a Y chromosome. Most men don't "do" hospitals well. Don't "do" illness well. Don't "do" caretaking well. I didn't plan for him to be any different, so I planned to do it without him. It was enough that he was footing all the bills. Would have a bald wife. Would watch the house fall apart while I ignored the chores for awhile. I knew he wanted to do it, but I made plans so he wouldn't have to do it. And deep in my heart, I knew I didn't want him to disappoint me or himself. What if he tried and couldn't? What if he started off fine and had to drop back? What if he didn't have what it takes in the hard places? What if it made him withdraw from me? I wanted to protect myself from knowing that about him.

Until he set me straight. This is happening to us, he said. I can't take the treatments for you, but I can be with you. I can't make you feel better but I can be with you when you feel awful. I can't make the decisions for you but I can make them with you. And my heart sang. And he did it. He did it better than any friend, any mother, any daughter. He was right in there with me, all the way. He never shrank, never got overwhelmed, never bailed out.

I had kissed a prince who turned out to be—a prince! And he didn't understand what had happened to all the other princes. Where were they?

While I was having treatment, he became concerned about a friend at work whose wife had been diagnosed with another cancer. He worried about him. A few weeks later, he came home furious. The husband was leaving. The marriage had been moving toward divorce anyway. The husband saw no reason to stay.

"How can he leave *now*?" my husband wanted to know. "What can be so bad that he can leave her to do this alone? What will their children think if he can split up with them *now* in *this*? Where is he?" he wanted to know.

I don't know where they are. I think some women want to do it alone. I think some women have to do it alone or with friends or sisters or mothers or daughters. I think some of them would do it but we push them away. My husband's oldest friend assured me at the beginning, "You think we can't do this, but we can. He can. This is a battle. Men are ready to do battle. He's not weak, he's been ready for this all his life. It's what will make him feel like a man. *The* man in your life. There's not a cowardly bone in his body."

I nearly made him a coward before he had a chance to do battle.

My mother would say, "You do this. It will only upset your father." "You come with me. This is too hard for your father. He has a heart condition, you know." I had come to think all of them had "a heart condition."

Now, I remember all the things I felt. He only remembers the process. Because the process is where he did battle for us. He still wants to hear from the men. He wants to know where they are. He thought he was part of a huge army. He feels as if he was really a sniper. He is looking for his regiment.

ARE YOU BETTER OFF WITH HIM OR WITHOUT HIM?
by Judy Klevins

"Thanks for leaving a message apologizing for your long message. It really made me feel better that you understand how hard it is for me to listen to such lengthy...well, it just over-whelms me when you talk so fast and long."

"Good."

"Well, how was your day? Mine was pretty good. I finally got the pump fixed at the farm. Thanks for helping with it last weekend."

"Look. I just can't chit-chat right now. I just walked in the door from the doctor's and a needle biopsy. They want to do a surgical biopsy on Monday."

"Oh, I'm so sorry. I hope you don't have to walk down that path."

"Could you drive me Monday?"

"Well, I don't know. I'll have to check. I hope things are O.K., but I really don't think it's fair that you call my day chit-chat. I mean, important things happened to me today, too."

My mother told me I always had to have a man around in case of an emergency. My man and a four year "committed" relationship unraveled during the diagnostic stage of my cancer.

Things were fraying before the lump was felt. I called him and left a message that I didn't want to see him that weekend. He never called again. I cried. When my friends found out, they needed to be restrained from telling him off. I reveled in their loyalty!

During treatment I was jealous of the women who had won-derful men with them. I thought that if only I were a better person, I too would have had a fine man with me.

Buried in one of the hundreds of articles and books I read on cancer was a liberating statistic: two out of every ten men leave a relationship when their woman gets breast cancer. They leave because they're scared, because they don't know what to do, because they realize they don't want to "walk down that path" with their woman, because of any number of reasons.

So I wasn't unusual. I had picked the wrong man and I was better off without him. I couldn't have gotten through cancer without the support of friends and groups. Finding the people who will help may take some time, but they are out there; it doesn't have to come from one place or person.

I CANNOT BELIEVE
by Lesley Tyson

i cannot believe
in the divinity
of forgiving
not for me
to pardon the deserters
i must be content
with the grace
of survival

SCHICK IT TO ME
by Rita Busch

Driving to the hospital for a breast biopsy, I realized I had not shaved my legs. I told my husband that I hated to go to a doctor with hairy legs. His reply: "If they're that far off target, you will have more important things to worry about than hair."

THE DARKEST MOMENT
by Daena Kluegel

He was so young, powerfully built with an athlete's muscled neck. He was trying to find that elusive vein to restart a "line," so he tried to help by chatting…"How's it going?"

"Pretty damned awful…. This waiting, when will I have the results?"

"Oh, I know about that."

"What do you know about that?"

In the twilight, as the room grew dimmer, he told me how he'd been ready to go to compete in the State High School Wrestling Tournament when he got sick. It turned out, he told me, that he was more than just sick. He had cancer, so when he "beat it," he decided to go into medicine and help others "beat it."

He left, reassuring me that it was "gonna be all right, I know it."

By that time, I was so thoroughly anxious that I could not relax. The "patient controlled anesthesia" had been restarted so I had no pain, but I felt terrible with the tubes and lines all over me and I felt alone with my overwhelming fear about the results of my node dissection. I was the color of baby food spinach. I had done okay during the first three days following my mastectomy. Shock, pain, and medication kept the thought process pretty frozen and paralyzed during that time, but now my thoughts raced in frantic turmoil. Questions raced through my mind: "Would I live to see my daughter graduate from college, my son married? Would I grow sicker and become a total burden on everyone?"

Another white coat entered and approached my bed. By this time, it was nearly dark and I was totally dissolved into self-pity and despair. The young man in the white coat had a sweet manner and was gentle and quiet but competent, and while he checked sutures, temps, drains, and wraps, he talked. He said that he'd decided to become a doctor following his mother's diagnosis and Halsted mastectomy for breast cancer. He saw how

CAN YOU COME HERE WHERE I AM?

the surgery had limited her in movement and in her life, (although he felt it did save her life). He vowed to help other women avoid that limit. He left with a sincere glance and said, "It will be all right."

By then, it was dark outside. I tried visualization. I cried. I prayed. I asked for healing from God. I tried to bargain with God. My heart was beating wildly, so fast that I thought I'd have a heart attack. What to do? How could I lie there and wait for the verdict?

Sometime about midnight, in the deepest black void, I decided that there was absolutely nothing that I could do to affect the outcome. In the old phrase of A. A., I "Let go and let God."

I felt a great calm. I felt peaceful for the first time since my biopsy three weeks earlier. My breathing slowed, the knot in my stomach loosened, and the lump in my dry throat shrank. Now I could almost feel my blood pressure dropping.

Then I slept soundly. The next morning, I woke to a sunny wintry day. After breakfast, (yes, I got it all down), the surgeon entered with his white-clad entourage. He was a very important surgeon so he had a large retinue. I recognized the two faces of my medical ministers from the previous night.

The surgeon was polite. "How are you?"

I was not interested in being polite or patient. "Any news?"

"Oh, yes, it's good...no positive nodes. You will want to discuss..." I never heard the end of his sentence.

After his exam and notes to the group, the surgeon left. The athlete smiled and winked as he left. The other young man lingered to say, "I knew because I saw the preliminary report but could not tell you; protocol, you know. I tried to tell you not to worry last night."

THE NUMBERS GAME
by Katherine Traynham

Forty-two percent of the women who have this kind will respond.

Eight percent of those will have to have this or that.

Twenty-two percent of women with your size tumor will need this.

Eleven percent of them will blah blah.

You have a one in eight chance of ever getting it. Oh, that's if you live into your eighties. For you, you hit a one in 700 chance, at your age. (Congratulations.)

If you also let us do this other thing, you'll increase your chances of living by another two percent. (Uh, is that two percent more of eight percent, eleven percent, or twenty-two percent? And is that of people who beat it completely, or for five years, or for ten?)

This is advanced math, that's for sure. Someone has written your name on a calendar. You always knew you would die someday. Or suspected it, anyway. There were years of calendars and on one of those blank days, you would die. That was bearable. Now it seems someone has written your name, in red, on a future day, in a specific month and year. It's the day you are going to die. But it's negotiable.

All the decisions you make at first will be based on *statistics*. How likely are you to die from this cancer? What are its dimensions? What was its exact location? How aggressive is it? What does it respond to and do you have any of that stuff in you? Now. Of all the women who fall in your general group, how many of them are dead? How many died in one year? Two years? Five? How many of them who had radiation died? Lived? When? How many who had chemo? What kind of chemo? For how long?

Now. Based on your kind of cancer, we pretty much know you won't die right away. If you do nothing, women like you die in this much time. If you have this surgery and this treatment, this many women, with your kind of cancer, who have this treatment, will live this long.

You make your decision based on the numbers. You want to be in the percent of a percent of the women like you who have what you have who do what you do and live. For five years. For ten years. For twenty years. For...oh, we don't have the statistics on that.

Once you start treatment, the numbers are still swimming in your head. You make your decision based on them. And one day you say to a doctor, "Well, I realize that percent of blah blah have etcetera happen to them." And the doctor looks at you and blinks and says, "Well, you can't pay any attention to statistics. That has nothing to do with you. You're an individual, not a number."

Now, don't you feel better?

STUPID PEOPLE TRICKS
by Daena Kluegel

After surgery and during chemo that spring at parent-teacher meetings, I had two very unnerving conferences with mothers of children in my classes. Each was a nurse and felt it important to make their actions and reasons for their actions perfectly clear to me in the conference. Since my Montessori program is a three-year program for three, four and five-year-olds, I teach most children for two or three years. These mothers had decided that they did not want their children in my class the next year. Each explained the reason in great and painful detail. They felt strongly that they did not want their young and fragile children to experience the death of their first teacher during the school year. They chose to put their three-year-olds in the other Montessori class at the school because, obviously, they felt that my fate was sealed.

I felt my face pale. My gut contracted painfully. My mind raced. "She thinks I'm going to die now or soon." There I sat at a table in my ordered classroom with a smile stuck on my face, hearing nothing past that stark declaration. My confidence seeped out through the scars on my chest.

I sat at each conference in total shock, barely able to mumble a polite reply, something like "thanks for your honesty." I wanted to scream at them, "So who made you God? How do you know that I won't survive the next year?" Instead, I went home and howled, cried and tried to rebuild my burst bubble of hard-won optimism about survival. Then, I wondered—had I ever done that to another person? God, I hope not!

I HAVE SURVIVED
by Lesley Tyson

i have survived
fire poison cutting steel
yet caught by unexpected reminders
the most bitter pain
is the self-inflicted torture
that comes with thoughts of you
when will my heart
be as numb to you
as my slowly fading scars

CHAPTER THREE

Bungee-Jumping Into
The Treatment Abyss

THE TATTOOS
by Helen Rash

On December 20, 1989, I began a chemotherapy protocol commonly called "CMF" (Cytoxan, Methotrexate, Fluorouracil). I never questioned my oncologist's decision on this or the radiation, because I had a great deal of confidence in his skills. At the age of twenty-five I had had ovarian cancer, and I had met him through this experience. In 1966 the only warning I'd had that anything was wrong was a little twinge in my side. I'd gone to him assuming it was something simple like appendicitis. He examined me thoroughly, ordered X-rays, and after viewing the films sent me immediately to a surgeon. By the time they removed the tumor, it was already the size of a small melon and was pressing on the organs around it. It was "encapsulated," which meant it had not metastasized to other parts of the body. I had no follow-up treatment and never had a recurrence. I know now I was very lucky. I've also learned since that time that many people would have recommended a complete hysterectomy, but my oncologist saw no evidence that this was necessary. In those days doctors often removed organs as a precautionary measure in situations such as mine.

I learned over time that the hallmark of my doctor's practice was that the patients' needs were paramount. This didn't always endear him to the nurses at local hospitals. He once decided that one of his patients wasn't receiving adequate care, so he picked her up and carried her to another part of the hospital and demanded that she be admitted there. And so, twenty-three years later, having grown up with this very bright man acting as my "case manager," I felt comfortable that we were doing the right thing. I was to have chemo every three weeks for six months, which meant ten treatments in all. A few days before each treatment I had to get routine blood work done to make sure I was ready to receive the next dose. There was only one time when the series was delayed because my blood wasn't strong enough. My early experience with these drugs was not at all what I had expected. I had no nausea until later on in the last few treatments, and my hair didn't fall out. I occasionally felt agitated and upset about being in treatment, however, these side effects were more emotional than physical. There were fluctuations in my body temperature, but these may have been related to other life changes I was going through at the time.

On my treatment day, I would go into my office and work in the morning and then drive almost an hour around the beltway to Maryland to my doctor's office, where his wife, a nurse, gave me the drugs using an IV drip. I know by talking to friends who've had chemo that I was fortunate in terms of how I was treated, both emotionally and physically. I sat in a lounge chair with my feet propped up and read magazines during the two hours or so that it took for the IV to finish. I listened to music on my little Walkman tape player or a radio. They gave me juice to drink and offered me candy to help take away the taste that sometimes comes with this particular set of drugs.

Afterward I drove all the way back to my house in south Arlington, often in the bitter cold and dark. I look back on that now as being almost irrational. I never thought of doing it any other way, and I believe also I was trying to prove to myself and to others that I could handle it. As soon as I got home, I would fall into bed and rest. Through trial and error I learned about the foods I liked during this time and began to prepare better for them. I seemed to crave bland foods, my favorite was a huge pile of mashed potatoes with sour cream and shredded cheese on top. I used instant potatoes and made things like Jell-O in advance so that I wouldn't have to cook.

Christmas 1989 was my first ever to be separated from family, but I'd decided that I could not fly to Illinois and risk wearing myself out with plane connections and perhaps bad weather. I was invited to be with friends on Christmas Eve and on Christmas day, and my niece flew out to spend New Year's with me. We got all dressed up on New Year's Eve and went to the Kennedy Center to see *Annie II*.

I had been told that the best time to buy a wig is *before* the hair falls out, so that the color and style can be matched better. Julie went with me, and I bought two wigs that closely matched my own hair. I put each on its little Styrofoam head and shoved them into the closet, not wanting to look at them with their blank white faces staring back at me. As it turned out, I never needed them and later donated both to the American Cancer Society.

I kept right on working during all of this, taking just my afternoon for treatment and then the next day to rest. On January 15, about three weeks after my first chemo, I began daily radiation for six weeks, Monday through Friday. My doctor had found me an excellent radiation oncologist at Alexandria Hospital just two miles from my home.

The radiation "simulation" (set-up) was a very stressful procedure, not because there was any pain, but because I had to lie absolutely immobile on a hard metal table for a very long time. The technicians, guided by the doctor, took a variety of very exacting measurements and marked on my chest with colored pens. The colored marks weren't to be washed off, since they were the road map for the technicians who would do the actual treatment. I was tattooed with a very tiny point like a fountain pen, which made a permanent black dot about the size of a freckle. These three dots were placed at the corners of the triangle of flesh at which the radiation would be directed.

The actual radiation therapy was certainly not difficult. I dropped by each morning at 8:00 and got the treatment, which took just a few minutes, and then went on to work. The clinic staff was young and supportive, and because we saw each other daily, we developed a kind of friendship. My skin turned pink, and I had to use a special greaseless cream to counter the burns. Other than this, I had no real side effects. My radiation oncologist was a wonderful, compassionate woman who was a little younger than I—easy to talk to, with a nice sense of humor. When I finished her set of treatments in late February, I had a fleeting sense of panic, which I found out later was normal. Having spent six weeks with kind and cheerful people in white coats *doing* something every day of the week to fight my cancer, suddenly, I was on my own again. Of course, I was glad to be finished, but I didn't know what lay ahead, except for the rest of my chemotherapy.

During early January I had called my former boss, the naval officer, and invited him for dinner. We had a very nice, relaxing evening, just eating and talking. I never saw him socially after that, but my two dates with him were very important to my recovery. Friends would ask if he'd called or kept in touch, and I would explain that it was O.K., regardless. I felt that I had been given this time with him just as a reminder that I could handle dating and that perhaps nothing had changed in that part of my life.

Toward the end of my chemo I did have some tolerable nausea, which would last for exactly twenty-four hours after the drugs had been given. Typically I would have dry heaves every hour regularly during that time. I convinced myself that this was not the worst thing in the world and that it would be over soon. I also reminded myself that women have similar problems during pregnancy, and they survive.

By June I began to have some real fears about my future, especially my relationships with men. I began to think no man would ever want me again, not because I'd had the surgery, but because they would be afraid my cancer would return. I felt "invisible" to men, and when I passed an attractive man on the street, I would lower my eyes...not a normal reaction for me. On June 24, I went for what I *thought* would be my second-to-last treatment, and my doctor told me that it was the last. I burst into tears, overwhelmed with a sense of relief. I'd forgotten that, due to the delay caused by a blood problem, we'd eliminated one of the treatments.

I'd never joined a breast cancer support group. There were two basic reasons: first, I couldn't say the word "cancer." I could say words like tumor, malignancy, medical problem, but "cancer" for me was a very loaded word. Secondly, I was worried that being with a group of women who'd had cancer might "bring me down." However, I had a chance to meet the social worker who ran the Arlington Hospital support group; and simply because I liked her so much, I decided to attend her meetings.

In July, 1990, I had a follow-up mammogram, which showed no problems. The head radiologist said, "You look fine. Go in peace." He also told me that the radiologist who'd discovered my tiny lump the fall before should be commended, since she'd done such a superb job of picking up on it. All in all, I was feeling very good and in general was so much happier than I'd been a year before.

THE SUN SHINES
by Lesley Tyson

the sun shines again
even in winter
i can still hope
even the cutting
poisoning
and burning
taste as much of life
as deeply desired
love and laughter

MYSTERY
by Daena Kluegel

I never thought I'd be involved in a murder mystery. Yet, here I am searching for clues and trying to be vigilant against the perpetrators. I know where they like to hang out and their "modus operandi." My team tried to surround and capture them at the scene of the crime. The team also spread deadly poison in case any of the gang got away and went into hiding at a distant location.

These "perps" are clever, vicious, dangerous, and downright malignant. The gang grows so fast and their activities are always underground. Even with strict surveillance, they cannot be safely contained. A regular Cosa Nostra, they are adept at infiltrating a quiet and innocent neighborhood and invading the lives of every inhabitant with catastrophic results. They are also terrorists. So when a test comes back with a slightly elevated result, I plan how I will deal with them, knowing they hold me hostage. I will bargain, I will fight, I will work with my team. I do not want to become the "corpus delicti."

PINK AND RED
by Jana Morgana

Pink and Red   In my paintings
In my decorations   In my clothes
Inside of Me
The inside of my body
Surgery   Drain   Clear tube
Pink fluid draining
A magnificent magical color
I swirl and twirl
I am pink inside   Alive
My body   Alive

NEITHER ONE NOR THE OTHER
by Katherine Traynham

It's the middle of life now. Not young, not yet old. You are no longer young and footloose, but not ready yet for the rocking chair, the wheelchair, or the nursing home. Suddenly, you moved into unfamiliar territory. You were healthy, felt great, did what you wanted. Now you're healthy, beginning to feel great again, and do even more of what you want. Somehow, though, you've moved into no-man's land. Can you say you're healthy if you've had cancer? If you've had chemotherapy and radiation? If they've cut into your breast and underarm and taken chunks away and analyzed it?

They got it all. You know that. The surgeon said so. (Do they ever say, "I think I left some bad stuff in there?" They always think they got it all, right?) You believe the best, but to be realistic, you're neither one thing nor the other anymore. Neither healthy nor sick. You're neither young nor old. You're neither dying nor fully living yet. You're neither carefree nor panicked. You were carefree once, then you were panicked. Now, you're neither one nor the other.

Your children were young once and needed a mother. They're not really adults yet, but almost, so you're not the mother of children, or the mother of adults. Your time to instruct and correct them isn't really over, but there's something wrong with you if you keep it up too much. You're neither one thing nor the other.

You still have your work, but you don't really feel the same way about it. Some days, you've been grateful for it and others you could hardly believe you ever wanted to do it at all. What were you thinking? So much has happened since your breast committed adultery with exactly the wrong kind of cell, you don't think you're who you used to be or who you'll be someday (presuming you live to get there), so you're neither one thing nor the other.

Is sex the same? Of course. Except. There's menopause. From the chemotherapy. You were looking forward to facing menopause gracefully someday. Not now. You would take hormones and calcium supplements. It would take a few years and then you'd be in the next phase of your life.

Only menopause for you lasted about three months, not three years. You raced right through that stage after the chemo killed your ovaries. You're not really an older woman now. You're certainly not any younger. But your body thinks it's through with middle age too, so that leaves you neither one place nor the other. Just about the time the kids left the house and you learned to enjoy sleeping naked again, all the regular juices stopped flowing. You want to be relieved. You want to act like it's no big deal—(compared to dying, it ain't)—but it's not your body anymore. It doesn't react the way it used to, you know. You need to have a little kick start in that direction sometimes. You weren't ready for diminished sexual desire. You weren't ready for an extramarital affair either, of course. You're just neither Lolita nor the Wise Woman. Maybe somewhere in between.

You don't concern yourself with the daily things your friends do. It's not particularly heartbreaking to hear about how they didn't get to buy the house they wanted, or their daughter didn't get into the college she wanted, even though four more accepted her. You want to tell your friends, "Big deal. Get over it. This is not a tragedy, take my word for it." You even want someone to tell *you* that about your cancer. You're not a cynic yet. You're also not Rebecca of Sunnybrook Farm anymore. You're neither a screaming harpy nor the pleasant grandmother type.

You didn't have a mastectomy. You're the beneficiary of breast-conservation therapies. You had breast cancer, and everybody wonders why you had chemotherapy if they didn't have to take your breast off. You aren't afraid to look at your breast in the mirror, but it isn't exactly looking back at you the same way. You're neither untouched nor seriously marred. Neither one thing nor the other.

You didn't turn out to be a coward. Of course, the symptoms from your treatment were mild compared to what they told you to expect. Your friends and husband were amazed. You looked courageous and uncomplaining. You were really just gritting your teeth and waiting for the other shoe to drop, but it never did. Then it was over. You wonder if you could do it if it were going to be worse. You're tempted to say you'll never do it again, anyway. You're neither brave nor a baby. Neither one nor the other.

It's not productive to feel sorry for yourself, so you don't. Most days, you even feel grateful—for life, for the people who love you, for the years you imagine you'll have stretched out before you. And then the suspense gets to you. You wonder if you're fatalistic. You wonder if the continuous testing isn't strain enough. Looking, always looking for more cancer, and praying it isn't there. And then in a few months, looking and looking again. It's not in your life or out of it. You wonder if there would be some sick relief in finding it. Getting the suspense over with. You think you're nuts for even thinking that, then you find out lots of women have thought that way. There it is again—you're neither crazy nor the perfect picture of mental health, are you?

There's really only one thing that you are without a doubt. Only one thing that doesn't take the neither/nor road in your mind right now. Only one thing that is a wholehearted *yes!* in this nether world of neithers. No one can say, "You're neither living nor dying." You may be walking between all the cracks on the sidewalk, eating but not enjoying, laughing but not being entertained, loving but not with abandon. You may be between a rock and a hard place, but you are still here. The heart pumps, the muscles flex, your eyes behold your beloved's and you can think and talk and read and comprehend and disagree and cry and blow your nose. You're alive and every breath you take is delicious. Every time you open your eyes (or shut them) it's the act of will from a living creature. You don't have one foot in the grave and one out of it, no matter what it feels like. You are absolutely among the living. You are truly alive. You are still here, still kicking, still on the roster, (maybe warming the bench), thinking about swinging for the bleachers, still hanging in there, still pulling the strings, still in the big time, still waiting for the fat lady to sing, still plugging along, still dishing it out, still soaking it up and you've definitely still got what it takes.

Oh sure, you still don't have any guarantees. Never did. But that's neither here nor there.

OH, FATHER!
by Rita Busch

BJ wanted to get a supply of Astroglide, a vaginal moisturizer, but learned that it was sold only in California at that time. No problem. She wrote her brother and had him buy it for her. Picture this man, a *priest*, in clerical collar, asking the druggist where he could find Astroglide!

RELEASE THIS VOW OF SILENCE
by Lesley Tyson

release this vow of silence
shifting paradigms
it seemed such a little time ago
i felt desperately challenged
by the wolf
a minor inconvenience
against that malignancy
that touched my womanhood
i continue alone
woman
whole in spirit

WHY ME?
by Daena Kluegel

Losses affect me bitterly. Losing a friend, a chance for a job or to improve myself distorts all of my life. Each loss is new and fresh, unlooked for, and I am never prepared or immune.

So, cancer, the diagnosis, treatment and subsequent changes are still bitterly resented by me. I will never again be able to trust and accept my body or its healthy functions. Now, I suspect due at least in part to my treatment, my body will never again function as before and I'm damned sure it'll never look the same. The hair did return but less full and lively—that's no great loss perhaps. The body is scarred and hugely out of symmetry as well as changed in mass by medicines to combat future death cells roving my reproductive system. Tamoxifen is still my best insurance against recurrence available to me. The loss of menstruation, of some sexuality, is all bitterly regretted. I am no Job, I still want justice, a reason. Why me?

Some of my early thoughts returned to guilt for actions or blame of my diet and lifestyle, but none of these was wildly different from the norm. Worse, with all the really terrible personalities around, why should I have this curse?

Then my daughter was diagnosed with lymphoma. She was finally starting a career in opera. At twenty-four, she was bright and healthy and lived a sedate and sensible life in order to care for her talent—her voice.

Bitterly, I searched for reasons, "Why, God, why?" What was the meaning or message? What about love and forgiveness and the innocence and purity of youth?

She suffered her long and intensive chemo-therapy...hairless, bloated and swollen, plagued by blisters and sores everywhere, unable to eat or sleep. I still am haunted by a vivid mental vision of her bent over a trash basket brushing out what remained of her lovely curly hair. I cried, she did not. And she was so brave! Her courage actually made me rage more. I remember what sorrow and anxiety I felt when she would no longer sing around the house. She had always sung. She sang before she talked. We always knew where she was, because we could hear her singing, even in her sleep. The house seemed to ring with the sad silence of non-singing. It was as if she had no joy or strength for song, needing all her strength in the battle for life and health, which was claiming all her resources. I knew that if she died, I would not go on.

It's so trite, but I really wanted to send the curse to pedophiles, drug dealers, terrorists and divert it from my child, my baby girl, but I was powerless to ease her awful agony. We are raised to expect that bad things will happen to bad people and I wanted justice now.

Well, we both made it. Changed, tempered and more able to meet misfortune with courage. It was no Gift, no Salvation, no Redemption. It was something which we rose to fight but never, never accepted. I felt that Primal Scream..."Why Me?" was mocked by the answer "Why not?" I still do not understand why bad things happen to good people, but I can testify that they do. I will always suspect anyone who counts Cancer as a "blessing." Madman, liar, or charlatan, it matters not. But do not burden me with your sermons and sympathies and pointless pontifications if you have never walked a mile in my moccasins, and most of you have not even put a toe in the shoe!

ROSE
by Katherine Traynham

My mother gave me a rose for my birthday.
A tea rose, Chrysler Imperial, blood red.
I planted it in the front yard
So I would see it, coming and going.
She told me red was for passion.
I'd just gotten married.
It bloomed every year, the most beautiful reds
On eighteen-inch stems
(From June to September.)

My mother gave me a rose for my birthday.
John Kennedy whites, pale and creamy and lush.
I planted it in the front yard
So I would see it all summer long.
She told me white was for memory.
Grandmother was gone now.
It bloomed every year. I fed it, and the red
(From June to September.)

My mother gave me a rose for my birthday.
The year after she died.
The year after my cancer.
I started in the front door as summer began.
It was May, and no roses came so early.
The white one had bloomed, of a sudden that night.
A single white rose on an eighteen-inch stem,
Even though I'd ignored them
(Last June to September.)

My mother gave me a rose for my birthday
The year I stopped loving roses.
The year after my chemo.
I saw its perfection despite my neglect,
And though I have never put stock in such signs

I took it inside and put it in a crystal vase
And showed my daughter what I didn't believe:

This rose shouldn't be here, in May, as I said.
(They bloom here from June to September.)
You feed them and tend to the canes when they're done.
I put them in the front yard, you know,
So you can see them coming and going.
And the John Kennedy white,—that's for memory.

My mother gave me this rose for my birthday.

BUMPS IN THE ROAD
by Helen Rash

Just before my mastectomy the surgeon had discovered some tiny bumps on my skin...each colorless, about the size of a mosquito bite and very innocuous looking. He said, "I know what these are, and I'll be able to remove them as I remove your breast." He called them skin metastases because they were an outgrowth of the malignancy. We gave them no more thought.

After the swelling from the surgery went down, however, there were about six remaining. These had been too far from the site of the actual incision to be recognized as a problem. They were still totally unobtrusive; and had I not been looking for them, they probably would have gone unnoticed. I showed them to my oncologist, who immediately got on the phone and called the doctor who had given me the radiation in 1990 after the lumpectomy. Now I was to go to her again for a consultation on these spots.

Unfortunately, on the day of my appointment she was away; and I was obliged to meet with her colleague, whom I'd never met before. Because my other experience with radiation had been rather positive, I went into this visit with a reasonably calm and upbeat attitude. It didn't take long for this to be dispelled. He kept using the words "at risk," as in "Those lymph nodes near your neck are at risk." I was devastated, terribly frightened. This time the series of treatments would last eight weeks, not six. The radiation would be focused on the *skin*; and because of this intensity, there was every chance there would be severe burns. But the worst news was that the radiation would probably damage my skin and toughen it so badly that reconstruction of the breast would no longer be an option.

I began to sob. He asked, "Are there any questions? Would you like to know anything about your prognosis?"

I was crying so hard that I couldn't get past a few words, which I kept repeating. "I don't...I don't..." Finally I got it out: "I don't deal in statistics. I don't want to hear them. They don't help me heal, and they don't make me feel any better." I had always believed that, short of someone telling me I had just a few months to live (and thus needed to get my affairs in order), I didn't want to hear any statistics. My oncologist, a very positive man, had never quoted me any data. Once, after my lumpectomy, I had asked him what the chances were that I might get cancer in the other breast. He said, "About one in ten."

Many women want to know all about their prognosis, and that's fine...for them. It had always been my contention that, if someone said I had a one in a million chance of surviving, there was no reason why I couldn't be the one.

Once again I found myself flat on my back on the hard metal table, with people drawing on my chest. I cried through the whole procedure, the salty tears running down my cheeks and into my ears. I stared up at the ceiling and vowed that life would hold more than this, that I would start writing my book; and, since I couldn't afford a computer, I would get a Dictaphone and begin recording the ideas on tape. Thus, the inspiration to settle down and finally begin writing was the offspring of my recurrent cancer and a determination not to be dragged down again.

The oncology social worker at the hospital was available to all patients, so I talked with her one day about my mastectomy and return to radiation. Because I was having to accept the possibility that reconstruction would never be an option, we discussed dating, sex, and how to disguise the fact that I had lost a breast. The crux of our conversation was that I should plan ahead, buying attractive lingerie or loungewear that I could keep on during the most intimate moments.

I embarked on the schedule of daily treatments in the fall of 1991 with the idea that this surely could wipe out half a dozen little skin lesions. Once again, like Gulliver surrounded by his Lilliputians, I lay on the table while people fussed over me. It was, in fact, very intense therapy. I did get burned so badly that occasionally my skin broke open. It took the full eight weeks and ended just as I was turning fifty-one...and at the second anniversary of the mammogram which had begun all this. We reached a point where we could find no evidence of cancer in my body.

Work had not been easy through all of the two years. I was working for someone who really lacked compassion, and there were days I simply dreaded the idea of any contact with my supervisor. Because I believed in the power of meditation, I added to my list of affirmations a statement about work and one about my boss. I began repeating: "I love my work, and I love my boss." This went on for a number of months until I realized that I didn't have to *love* either of them to survive. All I needed was to feel good about work and be able to have some kind of respect for my supervisor. So I just changed the key word to "like."

I also decided to experiment with another kind of imagery. I pictured millions of little Teenage Mutant Ninja Turtles inside my body, like tiny coal miners, hacking away at bad cells and dumping their lifeless forms into the bloodstream to be carried away. I have no idea why I chose these turtles, except that they had several good characteristics: they had a sense of humor, they were aggressive without being hostile, they were energetic, and they were green...a color which for me symbolizes growth, vitality, and harmony.

SIX DAYS OF COPING
by Helen Rash

A Diary

Sunday: Today my left arm, the one with the bad lymphedema, became very swollen and tender...all the way from my fingertips to my shoulder. I have no idea why. I've looked back over the last few days, and I know I haven't done any heavy lifting or anything to aggravate it. The lymphedema has bothered me emotionally more than my diagnosis of liver cancer five months ago. I know why, but it's hard to explain to someone who hasn't walked in my shoes: because I've survived cancer six different times in the last thirty years, I've begun to view it as "curable" or at worst "chronic" for me. On the other hand, this problem with my arms has no cure; I can manage it...bring the swelling under control...but I will have to deal with this the rest of my life. Also, I'd just learned how to select my clothes to cover my mastectomy scars, and now I have to deal with the cosmetics of this new problem. It doesn't seem fair.

This afternoon I spiked a very high fever, and I know I should have called my doctor. But I would like to have the weekends off from medical issues, just like I used to have them off when I worked. Several friends have called, and they've all scolded me for taking such a risk. This evening the fever went away...how strange.

Monday: Today at 9:00 I showed up at my oncologist's office and got good support from his nurse practitioner, who of course joined the chorus of scolders when she learned about my former fever. She gave me a prescription to take care of the infection. On the way home a tiny ant crawled across my windshield...I say tiny because he was no bigger than a grain of pepper. I turned on the wipers and sprayed him thoroughly with washer fluid, saying in my head, "Die, you fucking little ant!" I surprised even myself at this rage and then realized I had needed to get mad at someone but had no one to rail against. Poor little bug.

Michelle called, and I told her my story of the arm. After I hung up, I cried. Going further into my grief, I realized that prior to the edema, I'd always been able to disguise the fact that I'd had cancer. Now I had an outward symbol of the illness.

I ordered a compression sleeve to wear on my arm, and I guess that brought me one step closer to acceptance of something I can't control. Dave called to let me know how Mom was doing, and I talked to him about how I was feeling. Because he knows anatomy and other basic medical concepts, it's good to discuss these things with him.

Tuesday: I went to preschool today, and as always, it became my "happy pill." I've never known fatigue or sorrow during the times when I'm with those kids. Our little Pakistani boy, Assad, whispered to me, trilling his r's the way he does, "Miss Rash, can I show-and-tell you something?" Then he took me to his backpack and with great secrecy in his voice said, "Christmas is coming," and pulled out a Santa Claus ornament. I was sitting with Jonathan at one of the little tables, and he noticed how swollen my hand was. He touched it gently and said, "Why is your hand like that?" I simply told him it was sore. In a very fatherly, almost stern voice, he replied, "Then *why* are you in school today?"

Dave called, and I suspect it was just out of concern, since we'd talked yesterday.

Wednesday: Daena gave me a piece she'd written about her mother, who died just recently. Her mother was born with only one arm, and the writing was a tribute to this amazing woman, who taught school and raised children long before some of our modern conveniences, like diapers with Velcro tabs. It really helped me put things in perspective, and I made a mental note: next time I meditate, I must remember to say a thank-you for my two arms.

Charlann wrote from Phoenix. She'd read the essay Daena and I had written about how it feels when a friend gets cancer, and she said it helped *her* put some things into clearer focus. It's interesting how we give people comfort without intending to.

Tonight was writers' group. Since I no longer go to a support group, this set of friends has become a quasi-support-group and quasi-social-outlet. I know I can say anything I want to, no matter how clinical, so I shared what was going on with my edema.

Thursday: Today I cleaned house, since Diane and Al are coming for dinner Friday. It's amazing how bringing the house up to "company level" boosts my spirits...the smell of Windex, the polished furniture. Tonight I snuggled up in bed to watch my favorite NBC sitcoms and laughed out loud at "Seinfeld" as I often do. The cat curled up at my feet, as he always does. I'm sleeping better than I was a few days ago.

Friday: I went out and got my groceries this morning and tonight had a great dinner with D and Al. They've just returned from their trip to Florence, which was my favorite Italian city...and we sipped wine and had fun just talking and laughing. Today I thought of doing a little watercolor for D's grandchild, who'll arrive in early December...but then I realized that puts too much pressure on my time and energy...so I'll just buy a shower gift like other people.

NO PUKING ALLOWED
by Rita Busch

At the start of my next chemotherapy, my oncologist said, "How are you?"

"Fine," I answered, "but you're about to fix that, aren't you?"

LEAVING RAPPACCINI
by Helen Rash

There is a story by Nathaniel Hawthorne called "Rappaccini's Daughter" which began to flicker through my mind as I approached my twenty-first TAXOL treatment. The scientist Dr. Rappaccini has a lovely daughter whom he wants to protect from the evils of the outside world. Throughout her young life he exposes her to poisonous substances and plants, so that by the time she reaches womanhood, her very breath is capable of killing any living thing that is near her. Imprisoned and poisonous, she is allowed to roam the city streets, but her heart yearns for the sustenance of love.

I had the awful sense of being given poison which was keeping me alive...protected from the evils of the outside world. But I yearned to end the treatments and become normal again. This set up a great conflict within me. I had gone on TAXOL in March of 1993, just after it became available to the general public. In those days the drug was being derived directly from the bark of the yew tree. It was a twenty-four-hour-long IV procedure, so there were several times when I had to spend two nights in the hospital just to complete the treatment. I would leave work, check into the hospital and begin the protocol around supper time. If all went well, I'd be home the next evening. I learned to sleep with the IV in place and an automated blood-pressure cuff squeezing my arm at regular intervals throughout the night. Eventually the TAXOL scientists decided to reduce the number of hours required for the treatment, and I would simply sleep through the night and go home the next morning.

Two weeks after I began the treatment, my scalp turned fiery hot; and my hair began to fall out. I sensed that at some point I would want just to whack off the remaining hair and go ahead with a wig. So I laid out the wig and some scissors, waiting for that moment. It came after several days of fallout. The loss of the hair...the constant shedding...was in many ways more difficult than the final baldness. I've talked to a number of women who felt the same way. The drug was so powerful that I lost *every* hair on my body: eyebrows, eyelashes, pubic hair, and the soft peach fuzz we all have on our cheeks. I was still working at the time, and every morning I got up and drew on eyebrows and put eyeliner along the edge of my lids.

So I became this absolutely hairless person; and, since I'm very fair-skinned and rather slim, I often felt I looked like a little space creature. This cosmetic horror was briefly turned to good when I was asked to be a "model" and help train the beauticians who volunteered for the "Look Good, Feel Better" program of the American Cancer Society. I arrived at the training room without make-up and wearing only a beige turban. I wanted them to see what they might be facing as they helped women with make-up, wigs, and scarves. I briefly told them my story, and they practiced drawing in my eyebrows and putting various wigs and scarves on my head. They were amazed at what cosmetics could do for someone in my situation.

The TAXOL went on every three weeks for fifteen months. My old oncologist retired and sold his practice to a well-known oncology group in Maryland. I wasn't pleased with my relationship with the new doctor; but I stuck it out, assuming that at any moment I'd be done with the chemo and could change doctors. The treatment schedule fell into a pattern. I would see my doctor every three weeks, and he would simply give me orders for the hospital. We almost never talked, and I began to think he really didn't know what to do with me. The only active cancer I had was metastatic skin disease, and I believe he was afraid to stop treatment for fear my body would suddenly develop some life-threatening form of cancer. This attitude of his, coupled with my fear of ending the chemo, meant that we continued in silence.

I liked the two younger partners in the practice, and often they came to see me when they covered the hospital rounds. In June of 1994, one of them stopped by my bed. He said, "Well, how are you doing?" I began to sob. He asked, "When is the last time you and Dr. X actually sat down and developed a plan...and you remained dressed and participated in the discussion?" I told him we never had. He said that when his patients became frustrated, he knew it was time to do this. He recommended that I set up a "consultation" with his senior partner in which we would develop a plan. He told me to be sure to explain to the receptionist the reason for my wanting the appointment. And so I did. Meantime, however, I decided to go see a well-known oncologist in Arlington, Virginia, where I lived.

Before my consultation with Dr. X, I visited with this second doctor, whom I'd met through my support group and whom I liked very much. When he heard my history, he said, "Well, you never planned to be the poster-child for TAXOL, did you!?" (I think twenty-one treatments is probably a world record.) He told me what he would do if I were his patient, beginning with taking me off the chemo. He explained that if I continued, I might suffer organ damage; and he didn't believe my body would explode with disease if we stopped the treatment. I was amazed at how much we accomplished in our discussion, and I decided then to change doctors. When I had my official visit two weeks later with Dr. X, he had in hand a very carefully worded letter he'd received from the Arlington doctor. Dr. X, my own private Rappaccini, continued to talk as if I were his patient. Then I very quietly told him I'd decided to change doctors. To save him embarrassment, I said it was because I was tired of the long drive to Maryland.

HAIR TODAY
by Rita Busch

I didn't say "Why me?" or cry about the unfairness of getting cancer, but I did bitch and moan about the hair on my head falling out while the hair on my legs, underarms, lip, and chin kept growing. Now *that* is unfair.

THE HAIRCUT
by Katherine Traynham

This husband woke up in the middle of the night. His wife was out of bed and the bathroom light was on. He could hear her struggling and something clicking repeatedly. Then water running, then clicking again. He opened the bathroom door and she froze, scissors in hand, crying, trying to clip the last shreds of her hair. "What in the world are you doing?" he wanted to know.

She explained she was sick of the hair in her mouth, on her pillow, and in her food. It was worse falling out than being bald. She'd cut it as close as she could weeks ago, and it was still driving her crazy. If she could reach all around, she'd shave her head. He took the scissors out of her hand and began to clip the rest away.

"Thank God." He grinned at her. "I was afraid you were clipping the dog again!"

TEARS
by Daena Kluegel

When and why we cry or cried...
TEARS of shock. "No, not me, it's not true."
TEARS of realization of mortality, "What will happen to me, to those I love?"
TEARS of anger, "Why me? Pick on someone else who deserves it. Why has my body betrayed me when I did all I could to stay healthy?"

TEARS of guilt, "What did I do, how do I deserve this?"
TEARS of acceptance, "Let Go and Let God."
TEARS of compassion, "Another woman is now on that sad journey and may need my help."
TEARS of happiness, the discovery of life after this and how precious life is. Joy in sweet moments every day savored and cherished.

TEARS in certain moments of unlooked-for beauty and unexpected kindness which may be minor but has great impact and brings tears. When I hear my daughter sing or I see a rambunctious pup full of life and mischief, I puddle up. It can be inconvenient and can disrupt normal conversation. I am reminded of what Emily says in "Our Town" about life being too beautiful to be appreciated when we are living it. So I smile and soon the lump in my throat and the mist in my eyes clear and I'm almost normal again.

POISONED TEARS
by Katherine Traynham

I cry at anything. Everything. I cry at diaper commercials. I cry when my husband unintentionally hurts my feelings once every five years. I cry when I get mad. I get mad when I cry when I get mad, so I cry more. I cry when my daughter looks beautiful. I cry when I think about my mother, and that she is dead. I cry when I think about my father because he was never happy the way I understand it. I cry when disaster kills women and children. I cry when someone young has a terrible disease. I cry when I hear of a rape.

When the lump turned out to be cancer, I nearly choked on crying. Literally. It felt as if I couldn't swallow. It felt like needing to cry. I would cry and still feel the tears in my throat. I ate, swallowing over the choking. I went to sleep feeling the choke in my throat and I woke up with it. I wondered if I had cancer of the throat. I thought, maybe if I throw up it won't feel like this. I began to think the choking was something I would always feel. I did meditation. I did music therapy. I couldn't make it go away.

I had good reasons to cry. My mother died on a sunny September morning. We buried her and my ill father came home with me to live. I didn't cry around him except for one day when we cried together for six hours and talked about her. I felt I had responsibilities to him. If he wasn't crying, I couldn't let him find me doing it. He was seventy-six. Over the next four months, his health improved. Mine obviously got worse. He went home to live by himself for awhile. I started crying. I walked the floor and cried. I woke up crying. I went to take a bath because I could cry alone in there and wash my face without my family being suspicious. Three months later, my mother had been dead nine months. I had gotten through my first Mother's Day without her. Then I found a lump in my breast.

I wasn't choking yet. I wasn't choking during several needle aspirations. Or the ultrasound. Or the mammograms. I wasn't choking when they found a tiny cyst in the *other* breast I hadn't found yet. They got fluid out and that wasn't cancer, but the original lump was being stubborn. I wasn't choking when they put the IV in my arm for surgery.

I was choking when I woke up because I had briefly heard the doctor while I was "out" under twilight anesthesia. I heard him say, "I didn't want [or expect?] to find this." Or something like that. So I knew.

And through the recovery and the next surgery two weeks later. I was choking. I told them I was choking. They didn't know what to do for me. They didn't suggest anything. I was choking on fear. Is there a prescription for that? An operation?

I talked to a friend, a ten-year survivor of breast cancer. I said, "I feel like there's something in my throat." She described it to me. She knew exactly what it felt like. She said, "You may want to ask the doctor for something to make that feeling go away." I ignored her. I thought, millions of women have faced this and worse. Do they all ask for drugs to get through it? What did we do before there were these drugs? We gutted it out. I have to gut it out, myself, or I'll cover it up or something.

My husband took me to the doctor. He said, "Is there something you can give her?" The doctor wanted to know if I was depressed. No, I said. Not in a clinical way. I get up. I shower. I eat. I run errands. I write. I make the bed. I sleep soundly. I told him I felt impending doom. As if something horrible were about to happen to me. "It already did," he said, "This is anxiety. I'm going to give you an anti-anxiety pill."

I took the pills because I trusted my husband more than myself. Four days later, I stopped choking.

I started chemotherapy. Two weeks later, my sister called. Our father had died in his sleep. My hair was falling out and I was going to have to go bury him. We drove 660 miles. I had just given myself shots for five days because my blood counts were so low. We stayed at a hotel when we got there because the house was full with my sister and her kids, and I needed the privacy. I stood in the hotel room shower and my hair fell out in chunks. I would get out of the shower with wet hair covering me like Sasquatch. Softball-sized clumps of wet hair had to be fished out of the drain. I stood there and cried, not because of the hair but because I thought my father died because he couldn't stand it that I had cancer too, after Mom died from it. She hadn't been dead a year yet, so I cried for all of us. And my tears were sticky. They tasted like metal. My eyes would nearly glue themselves shut. I'd wash them and they still felt like honey.

This was the worst. Not the hair, not the effects from the chemo. Not the wig, not the general feeling of being exhausted. Not even the grief. The worst for me was that my tears felt poisoned. Not cleansing. Not warm and wet and salty. Sticky. Sickly. Gummy. I couldn't cry and feel better because every tear felt different.

They'd told me about nausea. About dizziness, skin changes, headaches, vision, and hearing loss. Tingling in toes and fingertips. Hair loss. They didn't tell me my tears would feel thick and bitter from one of the chemo drugs.

I didn't cry anymore. We buried my father. I went home. Chemo went fine. Four treatments were with Adriamycin. The next four would be with another chemical so I could have radiation as well. I didn't cry anymore for those three months. I wanted to cry for my mother, my father, myself. (Tell the truth.) Okay, I wanted to cry for me, first and foremost, and almost only. But I didn't know it. I went into private therapy. I cried and the tears weren't gummy anymore. I cried on the way home from the first session. I cried for five weeks. I cried so hard in one session I couldn't speak. I hadn't cried like that since I was a little girl. I found out what had been choking me. I didn't want my daughter to lose me like I lost my mother. The therapist said something that made me realize I wasn't crying for my mother. I was crying for my daughter and her mother. If it hurt so bad to lose your mother at forty-three, how would it feel to lose her at sixteen? seventeen? eighteen? I knew I would live long enough to see her graduate from high school in nine months. Would I see her graduate from college? Get married? Have babies? I cried for the woman who might have a baby without her mother around. I cried for the baby who might not have a grandmother. I cried for my daughter having to do it without her mother around. I cried for my not knowing what would happen to them. I cried because when my daughter dies, I won't be there to help. I cried because life is so crazy, she could actually die before me and I would be there and I don't want to be alive when she dies.

I cried because my husband is young. At forty-three, he would marry again. He would have twenty or thirty years with another woman. We'd only had ten. I cried because he would be with someone else three times as long as he'd been with me. I would be a distant memory. He might have children with another woman and we had only our children by different spouses. He would love another woman, longer, deeper, better than he had loved me. She would be the love of his life. I cried because my parents had been married for fifty-six years and they were buried side by side. I cried because I might be buried alone and my husband beside someone else. I cried because I would never know. He would be the love of my life, the kind in movies and books that is the heart of your heart, the singing in you and when you are old and no one can imagine that you could ever have been loved or loved that way, you always have that. And someone else would be that for him. And I hated her.

I cried because I was this weak and foolish. Because I was so selfish. I was crying for me and not my dead mother and father. I cried because cancer had taken a dear friend two months before my father died. She was only thirty-three. Her husband was getting married again. It hadn't even been a year. I didn't really cry for her. I cried because my husband might get married again before it had even been a year. I cried because none of this was happening to me and might not ever and I was crying because it *might*.

And then I was through.

Not with crying forever. But I was through with crying and crying and not knowing why and never understanding it and feeling worse instead of better.

And then, chemo was over. Radiation was over. Another Mother's Day came and went. My grandmother's sister died. She was 100 years old. She had wanted to die for a long time. I want to live for a long time. I cried, briefly. It was for my wanting to live, not for her dying. I called her grandson, my cousin. We talked about playing at her house in the summers. We would have his grandmother and mine—sisters—in the same house, doting on us. He cried for her, on the phone. I didn't.

I used to cry at anything. Everything. I was always crying for me.

X-RAY VISION
by Katherine Traynham

I could hardly drive myself there, every morning, for six weeks plus a day or two. The hospital had given me a parking pass, so I could park for free, close to the entrance. They were making it as easy as possible. I was gaining weight instead of losing, and I was unhappy about that, so they let me skip the Thursday weigh-ins. They were kind, compassionate, concerned.

And I dreaded it more and more every day.

It was supposed to be the easy part.

A few seconds, in a hospital gown, lying still, arm extended. A minute or two of a "zzzzzt!" sound and then get dressed and go home. They let me pick the time. Mornings? No problem. Lunch? We'll fit you in.

It wasn't when they did it. It was *that* they did it.

I was Miss Cheerful. I came in chatty, asking about the weekends they'd all had. I talked to people in the waiting room, admired knitting and needlework by women there with husbands being irradiated. I learned one of the nurses was raising her daughter's children, and asked all about how she was doing it. The younger technicians told me about their husbands and early Christmas presents.

I had cried all the way there, arriving early so I'd have time to fix my make-up. And then I'd get in the car, show my free parking pass to the gate attendant and, as I pulled away from the hospital, I'd cry all the way home.

My friends offered to go with me, as did my husband.

Don't be ridiculous, I told them. It's no big deal. It takes fifteen minutes to get there, six minutes start to finish once I walk in the door, and fifteen minutes home. I feel fine.

I honestly didn't care that my skin began to redden. I didn't mind that my breast was swelling a little. It was that every-day thing. Every day, first thing, I had to think: I have breast cancer and so I'm going to the hospital to have radiation. Every Monday through Friday for weeks. I loved the weekends. I woke up and thought, No Hospital Today. No machine noises. No hospital gowns. No lying on the cold table. No staring at the ceiling while the machines go, "Zzzzzzz…errrrrrrr…zzzzzzzzzzt!"

They leave the room while they do it. Radiation is bad for you, so they leave the room. Radiation is bad for you. Unless you need radiation to kill something worse, like cancer.

Every day. Monday through Friday. For six weeks, plus a few days. Cooking your breast until part of it is bright red and tender. Microwaved.

It's no big deal. It doesn't hurt. It's the easiest part. It keeps the cancer from coming back—in that breast (you hope). The technicians are nice. They give you brochures and ask if you want to meet with a nutritionist. (No.) They give you handouts about their support groups. (I already don't want to come here every day, so I should come here at night, too? I don't think so.) You can bring a CD or a tape and they'll play it for you while you're lying there.

Why did I cry every day? Why did I get the shakes coming and going? Why do I hate to lie down on the table at the doctor's office now? No one is going to leave while machines microwave me and go "zzzzzt."

Don't leave me alone again, wearing a hospital gown, lying on a metal table, in a room with machines and a little butterfly decal to look at on the ceiling, while you close the heavy door and I wait, very still, for ninety seconds, while the machine you're afraid of buzzes. You don't have any idea what I'm seeing while you're in the other room.

I went to a gynecologist once. Actually, I go to one regularly, but this one only once. I sat on the table, in a hospital gown. He came in and so did his nurse. I lay back on the table and there, on the ceiling, was a pin-up of Tom Selleck. The nurse had put it there. Ha-ha, she said. It will give you something to think about. It certainly did. I thought about the phone book and how I would look under "Physicians: OB-GYN," as soon as I got home.

I looked at the butterfly while I was keeping my arm so still, getting my breast irradiated. Was I supposed to think happy thoughts? Practice "focal point" meditation learned in old childbirth classes?

Think about metamorphosis and what I was going to become? (No, thank you.)

The last day of radiation, I didn't cry on the way home. I hadn't left the hospital. I had escaped.

NECKLACE
by Judy Klevins

Fondling all Nordstrom's offers on their first floor
I hit the rack of celestial sphere necklaces

When the metallic racket subsides
One pillowed heart swings out
Making sweet angel sounds

My world is falling apart
Sewers back up
Termites infest my house
The Honda dies
Cancer cells and radiation rays run through my body

Not one more thing
Not one more thing

A small perfection
A chiming heart on a long silver chain

Finds me

Keeps hope alive

ALMOST UNACKNOWLEDGED
by Lesley Tyson

almost unacknowledged
another dark anniversary passes
moving at light speed
pushing through the wall
once or twice stopping to rest
the drugged oblivion of that moment
gently surrounds me feather light
as the faint body deep memory
tentatively touches my thoughts
survival is almost the only answer

UNCERTAIN
by Lesley Tyson

uncertain
how to measure
the time left
wanting infinite days
that may too easily be counted
just know
and live it all as a lifetime

WHEN
by Katherine Traynham

Somewhere near the next-to-last chemo, I began thinking of myself as someone who had cancer. I had stopped being so surprised at what was happening to me. I had been well, but worn out from what was going on in my life. Then a doctor said I had cancer and all of a sudden, I was struggling to comprehend because I wasn't "sick." No symptoms, so how could I have cancer? Cancer is the diagnosis you get when you have weird symptoms for months and months and you trudge from doctor to doctor and they don't find anything. Finally, you go to a specialist, and he names it for you: cancer.

I didn't need a name for anything. I wasn't looking for a reason why I had blood in my urine or strange pains that kept me in bed. I was fine. Honest.

I still felt that way for a long time after treatment began. The hair loss, weird bloating, dark circles under my eyes—that wasn't the cancer, that was the treatment I was taking to kill off the cancer. I still wasn't sick—just temporarily indisposed.

I don't know when it changed. One day, I looked in the mirror and wasn't shocked by the changes anymore, I guess. It wasn't someone odd staring out at me. It was me, and I recognized her. That's what I looked like. I began humming, "I've Grown Accustomed to Your Face," as I did my make-up and painted on eyebrows where there were none. I had begun to think of myself as "someone who has?/had? cancer." And worse, I began to act like it.

I wanted everyone to know that things were different now. And in case they hadn't made the connection, I made it for them. "Well," I'd sneak into a perfectly innocuous conversation, "I felt that way, too—UNTIL I HAD CANCER!" See, everything is different after cancer. There were those who hadn't had it and didn't know how different the world was—and then there was me, and everybody who'd had cancer, and, well...we just *knew*, that's all. It's as if everyone *not* on the Cancer Enlightenment Program was slightly retarded. It couldn't be helped, you see. They just had no idea. Poor dears, they were tripping through life lightheartedly, like children playing in a minefield. They were bound to step on something that would blow them up eventually. I, the old soldier, stood at the edge of the field, tsk-tsking and constantly pointing to my artificial leg and Bronze Star. They needed to grow up and grow up fast. What a pain I became.

Plus, it was boring. Even I knew that. And because I had chosen this position for myself, I forgot that it would change. The symptoms from chemo abated. Slowly, slowly, my face began to look like the old face. I looked more like me than I ever thought I would again.

I began to think about living again. Not for twenty years, but maybe for twenty more months. Maybe this stuff was going to take me out, but it didn't seem to be taking me out very fast! Despite my feeling that I might die any minute, and certainly before I wanted to, it looked as if I would live until fall. Christmas. Spring. Oh, heck, maybe till next Christmas.

Before I knew it, I was living again. And millimeter by millimeter, I began to be less tired. I wondered if I might feel young again someday. Or care about the spot on the dining room rug. I wondered if I might one day watch the news and not feel so deeply, deeply sad for the whole world. Or push myself to finish everything—this week, because who knows how much time we have anyway?

I still didn't want to talk about the future. The future was for those poor people who didn't know—who hadn't had the crash course in Cancer. My husband often talked about Italy—laughed and said he was afraid for us to take a trip there, because he just knew we would love it so much we'd never return and have to have the furniture and dog shipped to us. I got the shakes when he would say that. I didn't have any castles in the sky left, so how could I dream about villas in Italy? Didn't he know "someday" was for people who had futures?

And one day, enough was enough. We sat down to talk about money, just before our oldest daughter's second semester in college began. We finished that and did some calculations for what we would have had if we'd put away 100 dollars a month from the day she was born. Then we figured out what we could reasonably do for her by the time she turned twenty-eight. I laughed and made a joke (I thought). I said it would be easier if I just died and she'd get more money that way.

"Don't say that," he said as he turned away.

It wasn't funny, was it? And so I was finally through. I had been a coward for a year since my treatment ended. I had reminded everyone that I was exempt from the future because I might not be here. Not *wouldn't* be here—just *might not* be here. I wasn't willing to play the "Someday, what if?" game because it might not include me. And so I said something stupid to my husband, just in case he'd managed to forget for twenty minutes.

I'm through now. No doubt I'll still have moments when I don't trust the future, sweat my next checkup, think the next freckle or cough is cancer—and it might be. But I'm not going to live that way every day and make everybody else leave me out of their plans because I'm afraid of the disappointment if I don't get to go into tomorrow with them.

I'm through and I'm going to live. Every day. For a long time. I don't care that I don't know how long it is, because nobody does. They just don't know they don't know. And I'm glad they don't. I'm going to live and I'm going to Italy and I'm going to grow old and my daughter will be very old before she gets any insurance money out of me. And if something stops me, I'll have time to grieve when I get there. I don't have to hold Dread's hand every step of the way. Sorrow can wait for a reason for sorrow. Joy is the order of the day. When? Starting immediately.

PESKY DANDRUFF
by Katherine Traynham

My hair was gone now. My family was so kind, so sweet about it. My husband touched me and held me and offered to shave his head, too. But both he and my daughter watched me. Constantly. When they thought I wasn't looking. One Saturday, they furtively studied me as I puttered around the kitchen. Finally, I turned to them with their serious eyes, rubbed my slick scalp and said, "Well, I guess I've finally cured that pesky dandruff problem!" They fell out of their chairs laughing and stopped studying my every move.

HAIR AND NOW
by Rita Busch

During chemotherapy, I was horrified to find that a facial depilatory caused burning and rash and for the first time, I could do nothing about my dark mustache. I complained to my surgeon that over the last few months, I'd had to ask my husband: Now that I have a large scar from having my gallbladder removed, do you still love me? Then, Now that I have a gallbladder scar and only one boob, do you still love me. Then, Now that I've lost most of my hair, have only one boob, and a gallbladder scar, do you still love me.

So, now I have to say, With only one boob, scars galore, no hair on my head, and a damned mustache, do you still love me?

YES, I SAID THAT IN SUPPORT GROUP
by Daena Kluegel

I realized how fatal this thing can be and said to myself as I watched my son playing with his year-old puppy, "Oh no, I might not outlive that pup." Then, I decided to buy no new clothes for a year as I might not live long enough to wear them. Sometimes, I put myself and my anxiety under limits: "I lived through that test, I can live until the next round of tests or Christmas or Easter." Recovery is a long and hard process. At first I only wanted to get the tumor out of my body, then I wanted to kill any rogue cells. Using surgery and chemotherapy, we did as much as medicine knows to do to accomplish these tasks but then I had to learn how to live with this knowledge that my body had betrayed me once. I had to learn to live with anxiety and uncertainty which for me, a control freak, is a Herculean task requiring major restructuring of mind processes.

I dislike the word "remission" because it implies return. This is waiting for the other shoe to drop. Still, it is a much less fear-laden word than "metastasis" or "recurrence." It is hard to maintain life only day by day with no thought about the future. Sometimes it becomes exhausting. It is difficult to have energy for what life throws at you when you are constantly beating back the dark fear lurking in the corner of your consciousness.

One day you realize that you haven't thought about IT for ten minutes. Sometimes you can even go thirty minutes without IT preoccupying your thoughts. IT no longer envelops you, wrapping you and all your thoughts in ITS tenacious grasp. Every ache, every hangnail no longer brings thoughts of metastasis, with trips to the symptom list in the CANCER Book. You bargain yourself out of panic: "If it's worse or no better in a week, I'll call the oncologist." You plan your memorial service as you drive to have a follow-up mammogram after having a post diagnosis "bad" one.

Your life is now demarcated as BC and AD. That is Before Cancer and After Diagnosis.

CHAPTER FOUR

It's Over Already?

MODELS
by Helen Rash

"I really like your hair."

"Thank you. For the first time I'm wearing it really short."

I could hardly contain myself. The registrar at the Wolf Modeling Agency had just paid me a compliment on my hairdo, and only I knew that the cap of auburn curls was just an outgrowth after chemo. My hair had grown in naturally curly and slightly darker than my strawberry blonde "pre-chemo" look. My hairdresser had added some coppery tones, and the overall effect was rather sassy and youthful.

Exactly one month before my visit to Wolf, I'd had my second breast removed...a prophylactic mastectomy which I'd willingly scheduled. My doctors fully supported me, knowing that cosmetically I'd felt out of balance, and that, given my history, I'd always be waiting for the other shoe to drop. What we *hadn't* known was that the breast contained malignant tumors, and so I really dodged a bullet.

Because I'd had so much surgery and radiation, I was worried that my posture would start to slip and that I'd develop a defensive way of walking and sitting. And so I decided to go to modeling school, not to become a professional, but to focus on my appearance, wardrobe, and general attitude about my body. Beginning in high school I'd been interested in make-up and skin care, but I thought I could pick up some tips in the modeling school sessions. That's how I came to be sitting across from the registrar, smiling my secret smile. I signed up for the full twenty sessions, one each week on Thursday nights.

Before we got into the basics of runway walks and turns, we had to go through several classes on things like nutrition, weight control, and what might best be described as "charm school." In the nutrition and diet session I had to have my measurements taken and recorded by several fellow students, all about fourteen years old. As it turned out, the average person in the school was between fourteen and twenty-four and had flawless skin. I began to feel like a sorority housemother, but I actually enjoyed it. The kids were very nice to me. One little eleven-year-old said, "Are you in *college?*" I loved that.

My greatest reward for all this was that I had a place to go where no one uttered the word "cancer," and no one knew I had no bosom. We had homework assignments which the young girls never bothered to turn in, but which I faithfully carried out. One was to go through magazines and catalogs and pick out clothes we liked and which suited our particular style. I diligently clipped and glued pictures in a scrapbook. What I learned from this exercise was actually quite valuable. My body had been under assault for five years, and I'd begun to think that pretty clothes were going to be a thing of the past. As it turned out, I found great turtlenecks, mini skirts, boots, and other things I really liked and that were figure-flattering.

When the modeling series finished, I went on to take ten acting classes. Before each class we did stretches and physical warm-ups to loosen our bodies. This supported my original reason for taking the acting lessons: to learn to speak with my body again. I'd spent most of my life singing and doing public speaking, and I didn't want to lose those skills. We had to memorize and give monologues, so I chose two that were very different: Emily's farewell in *Our Town* and one of Lady Macbeth's more evil speeches.

What I took away from the modeling and acting was that I *could* get outside myself and that I could communicate with my body, in spite of the damage.

Not long after that, I awoke one Sunday morning and began to sob. I knew right away what was wrong. There were things I'd never been willing to say aloud to myself or anyone else...not even in support group. I had to admit that, had the devastation of my body taken place at the hands of an enemy, we would have called it *mutilation*. But because the surgeries and radiation were done by compassionate physicians, I was somehow supposed to buy into the idea that it was for my own good. I remember when I first joined a support group and had only a small scar on my breast, one woman had said she felt mutilated. Those words shocked me, but I would eventually come to understand what she meant. By Sunday evening I was back to normal, and on Monday I was downright perky.

LITTLE PURPLE BOTTLE
by Helen Rash

Dave, my brother, put a Ziplock bag filled with warm water in the bottom of a small cardboard box, creating a kind of hot-water bottle for the kittens. They had just been born by Caesarean section, and the mother, a tailless white Manx, was in her carrier, right next to the box. Her head bobbed from side to side, eyes still trying to focus after the anesthesia. The lower half of her body seemed to be made of lead. She couldn't move it.

My niece and nephew, Julie and Tom, and I had run across the driveway to the clinic as soon as we found out that the little cats had been born. With childlike awe, we peered down into the box as Dave took each of the four babies and put it in on the diaper that covered the warm sack. They were blind, damp, mewing, and they all had tails. Since the owner had hoped for a litter of tailless kittens, Dave would have to talk to him about the odds of having cats without tails when neither the mother nor the father was purebred.

While we were waiting for the client, we leaned on the stainless steel table and listened to the box making its tiny me-owing noises. Dave and Tom started to laugh about something which was clearly an inside joke. Dave reached up into the supply cabinet and pulled out a bottle with a bright purple label, raised it high, and said "If I ever get difficult and neurotic, I want you to remember where this bottle is." It turned out to be the fluid used to put dogs to sleep. We all giggled.

The next day was Christmas Eve, 1994. That day the client had to come back with the mother and the litter, because the cat had rejected her little ones and was hissing instead of nursing. Dave gave the mother cat something to calm her down. If that didn't work, the owner would have to feed them all by hand. A few days later, Dave took me as his guest to a rotary meeting, and on the way I asked him if he knew what had happened to the kittens, now five days old. He said he didn't really know, and that it was better if he didn't dwell on the fate of the kittens, since it was hard to do good vet work if he worried about each animal he brought into the world. I really understood what he meant by this.

* * * *

I wish I had my own little purple bottle. I would just put it way at the back of my closet in case I ever needed it. Anyone who has led a rich life, as I have, and faced the possibility of a debilitating or fatal illness can probably relate to this idea. It's not death I fear, but the image of being totally helpless and in pain. There was a woman named Mary Ann who came to our support group for a while, and suddenly she stopped coming. She'd had a difficult time of it, being told every few years that her cancer was back. The last time we saw her, she and her husband had just returned from a nice vacation in the Caribbean, and she seemed on top of things. Then he called our social worker and left a message, saying that she had died, and he wanted to donate all her clippings and books on cancer to our group. When Kathy finally was able to talk with him, he said that her doctors had told Mary Ann that they had nothing new to offer her to control the cancer. She despaired, sat down with her family and told them she didn't want to live. Then she took her own life.

I cried when I learned of the death of Lewis Puller, the Pulitzer-Prize-winning author of *Fortunate Son*...a Vietnam war hero who had lost both legs and parts of both hands in the war. For a long time he battled addiction to alcohol and painkillers and then one day just couldn't fight any longer. My reaction was, "I wonder how many times a person can keep going to the well of resilience and personal power before the moment when they finally decide the well is dry?" Of course, I knew that the moment would be different for each person, depending on so many factors. Just at that time a man I worked with died of a brain tumor, and on the program from his memorial service was a quote; "We are afflicted in every way, but not crushed; perplexed, but not driven to despair; persecuted but not forsaken; struck down, but not destroyed...." (II Cor. 4:8, 9)

There was an article in the *Washington Post* which talked about a study that had been done showing doctors have different reasons for deciding that further treatment is "futile." The article stated rather coldly that there were many reports on "quantitative futility" that suggest doctors make every effort to save the patient if the odds of survival are greater than one percent. Some studies indicated that doctors had written off patients that actually had a twenty percent or better chance of survival.

All of the statistics become so meaningless when they're applied to a real person, someone who has ideas about what life ought to hold for them. It's actually easy for me to be matter-of-fact right now about wanting to take my own life rather than suffer and become a bony, pale, tired person. This would not be "life" for me but just a dreadful holding pattern until my spirit can be released. But I won't dwell on this, because it's hard to "do good work" if one thinks about death too much.

SCREAMING
by Lesley Tyson

screaming
in silent disappointment
the determined belief
in the lifetime reprieve
proved so fearfully short
return to a full life
detoured again
not wanting
the rest of life
to be battles and pain
that distant shining light
stimulating courage
perhaps to find
a sweet life
amid the obstacles

A TRAIN TOO FAST TO CATCH
by Helen Rash

Some friends took me to lunch at a beautiful outdoor cafe in Scottsdale. The air was dry and fresh, and we had a great view of the mountains. An attractive older woman strolled through the tables, modeling some handmade vests. It was March, and I was very aware that if I had been back home, the weather would probably have been very unpleasant.

Afterward we went to the Spa at Camelback Inn, where we were signed up for various luxurious activities. Mine was an expensive facial. The interior of the spa was quietly elegant, and people spoke in soft tones. I went to the desk and was given a white terry-cloth robe, a cap, and a pair of paper slippers. Suddenly something flashed through my mind, like a train that goes by so quickly you can't even see the faces in the windows or read the print on the sides of the cars. This image lasted perhaps one second. I really didn't know what I'd seen.

We went to the women's locker area, and I chose to undress in a private booth rather than shock the other guests with the scars on my chest. Flash...flash. The *train* went by again, and I felt a heaviness in my body but still didn't see any details.

The next step was waiting in a lounge where other women with freshly painted toes and fingers chatted among themselves, and a TV droned in the corner...no one seemed to be watching. The women wore no make-up, and their heads were covered in towels or caps. Flash...flash...flash.

The esthetician who was to do my facial came to get me. She was middle-aged, wore a white dress and spoke with a foreign accent, perhaps German or Dutch. She gently led me to a room and asked me to wrap my body in a large towel, leaving my shoulders and neck exposed. Then I was to climb up on the table. Flash...flash...flash...flash.

She returned just as I began to sob. I explained that I'd lost both breasts. She was very kind. But I still didn't get it.

Flash...flash. The *train* suddenly stopped, and I stopped crying. What I saw was a string of pictures...people handing me

CAN YOU COME HERE WHERE I AM?

gowns to put on. People telling me where to wait. TV sets in the corner of lounges with no one in particular watching them. Women with soft voices wearing white uniforms telling me to climb up on the table. I hadn't given her the real explanation for my emotion. I'd given her the easy answer...that I was scarred. There was no need to tell any more, because now my eyes were dry, and I was enjoying the massage on my neck and shoulders.

THE NEWS
by Lesley Tyson

the news
not malignant
but not quite normal
it is enough
to know
that the enemy
has not returned
i will survive
for my yet uncounted days
and vigilance
like breathing
will become a habit

THE FIRST CHECK-UP
by Katherine Traynham

Treatment's over. You got a little break where you didn't have to see a single doctor for a month or two. Now it's time for your first mammogram since—well, since cancer. You go to the same place you always did. The same place as last time. The same place where they did the ultrasound. You took them your films because you've been carrying them from doctor to doctor for months. They can have them back now—everybody's pretty much memorized them, including you.

You're in that room—not the same one as last time, but the one next to it. You're wearing the gown, the machine is right there. You wonder if it will hurt this time. You never dreaded it before, but everything's different now.

The technician comes in. She'd like to ask you a couple of questions first. (I guess she would, considering what's been going on in your life!)

Then she says, "Have you had any symptoms since your last mammogram?"

You start laughing. You think, "She has got to be kidding, right?"

"Uh, symptoms?" you say.

She thinks you don't understand what she's looking for. She elaborates: "You know, anything different since you were here a year ago?"

Then you realize: she hasn't even opened your chart. This is a place that does hundreds, maybe thousands of mammograms. They are looking for cancer. Don't they have a sticker or special color folder or something that says, "Yep. Found it!"

Now you're mad. Yes, you guess you have had a few symptoms since you were here last. Does she mean since the two surgeries that came on the heels of the last mammogram? Or the spaced-out feeling during chemo? How about the condition of your skin during radiation? Is that what she's looking for?

She's turning pale now, but you go on. And then there's the part where you have stabbing pains off and on in the treated breast. Maybe that's a symptom? Or that your hair fell out and you gained twenty-five pounds? Could she be more specific? You just don't know which symptoms to mention. The weakness in your right arm? The cramping? That's almost gone now, so maybe it doesn't count.

You're starting to feel mean now, because she is clearly humiliated and you don't care. She doesn't dare open your file now, even though she's still holding it. Clearly, it says stuff in there about your cancer—all the other doctors sent copies of the continuing reports. You know, because you called to make sure they'd arrived.

She's stumbling over her words now. She's looking at her little checklist.

"Um, okay. But no nipple discharge or anything like that?"

You smile. Nope. Haven't had that one yet. But if you do, you'll be sure to call. And then she says she'll be right back.

When she comes back, you're feeling evil. Okay, so she didn't read your chart before she walked in. She's probably twenty-three years old or something. Most of the women she sees *don't* have breast cancer, thank God.

She does the mammogram. She's very careful. Very gentle. For some reason, it irritates you even more. The doctor comes in. He greets you warmly. He clearly remembers last year and that your nodes were negative and he celebrates with you that one happy note you cling to. Everything is fine now. See you in another year, unless something "comes up" sooner.

You get to the car and you can't drive for a few minutes. You're shaking from anger. Or about to cry.

Why don't they just read the damn chart?

WHERE'D SHE GO?
by Katherine Traynham

Suddenly, you realize you haven't heard from her in awhile. Like, since you were diagnosed with cancer. You called and told her the day you got your diagnosis. While you were still in that awful, awful panic. She told you to call a mutual friend who'd had breast cancer. You don't know why you didn't think of that. You were grateful she'd mentioned her. That's the last time you talked to her.

There were dozens of friends who came through for you. People you didn't even know felt they were your friends. You were overwhelmed and humbled that they cared for you and that they cared so much.

She wasn't one of them. Or, at least, wasn't one who could stay close by and show she cared. One day, you ran into her in the grocery store. She was clearly embarrassed. You looked fine, had gained some weight, had the wig on, but you were clearly not wasting away somewhere in a dark nursing home or hiding yourself away during treatment. She was flustered. She apologized a million times for not calling. You just wanted to chat and know how she was doing. She couldn't do it. She couldn't talk about the kids and resume where you'd left off. She had guilt written all over her face and if you said, "Look, don't feel guilty about bailing out on me," you would have made it worse. She didn't know you didn't have those expectations.

I HAD IT
by Jana Morgana

I had Breast Cancer
Societies Fear   Cancer
The Worst Thing
My fears   The medical establishment
My Body   Making a bad malignant thing
Is it my fault   Did I make it happen
Dazed with shock and fear
I moved ahead
I chose Doctors and treatments
I went through lumpectomy
Node testing   Radiation
Supported by children
Sister   Friends   And Groups
I cried   Shook with fear   Rested
I have done it   Lived a year
My Journey   Feeling the fear
Taking action
Seeing who I am
Softer   More relaxed
I have and can find
What I need for my life

CHAPTER FIVE

It's Never Over, Is It?

SLINGS, ARROWS, AND A THOUSAND NATURAL SHOCKS
by Helen Rash

During the fall of 1990, my *left* breast very gradually enlarged and became hard, and the nipple slowly inverted and disappeared. My oncologist referred me for an emergency mammogram just four months after my last one, but the results were inconclusive. We also tried using a sonogram, but this was also of no help. I then went to see my surgeon, who said I needed a biopsy immediately. We set it up for three days after Christmas. I also went to see my acupuncturist; and when he gave me a treatment on the meridian related to the breast, I felt something akin to an electrical shock.

In this same period I decided to drop out of my support group...at least for a while. Several women who had joined recently were having what I perceived to be a very negative impact on the group. They were bitter and angry, and the women seemed to be spending too much time simply recounting old problems rather than getting on with the development of coping skills. This sense of unease was coupled with my own ice-cold terror at the prospect of having cancer in my other breast just five months after ending chemo. I just couldn't sit and listen to other people's stories of misdiagnosis and physician insensitivity.

I told my acupuncturist about my congested left breast, and he suggested I rub it with boiled sesame oil, just in case it was not a malignancy but simply a routine treatable blockage of some kind. I went to Illinois for Christmas, and I spent a lot of time meditating, rubbing in the oil, and being terribly frightened.

The biopsy was Friday, December 28, 1990. The night before the procedure I stayed with Pattie, and in the morning I walked to the hospital, about five blocks from her home. We'd had a heavy snow the night before, and the walk in the cold, crisp air felt good and helped clear my head. My surgeon made a tiny incision just below the nipple. For the results of this biopsy I would have to wait until Monday. I returned to Pattie's house, and that evening we sat and talked and watched TV together. I bundled up in a huge purple velour robe that Dave and Louise had given me. I felt fairly relaxed, still believing they would find nothing.

On New Year's Eve day, I went to see the surgeon for the results. Once again it turned out to be cancer, but a different type from what had been found on the right side exactly a year before. He said I'd probably be given radiation or chemotherapy. I misunderstood, noting he didn't mention a mastectomy, and assumed I was headed for something fairly simple. I was wrong.

That evening Pattie and a friend and I spent New Year's Eve at the mall at Union Station, where hundreds of people milled about in party hats, drinking and blowing loudly through those little paper tubes that snap out and roll back again. I went through the motions of eating supper and making conversation, grateful that I had friends to be with. On New Year's Day I wrote in my journal that I'd hit a *glass* wall (not a *brick* wall, because that would imply that I'd seen what was coming).

I began focusing my meditations on three goals, in the form of three affirmations. In effect, I was trying to program myself to achieve the things I wanted most in life, even though they seemed to have eluded me:

- My days are filled with joy.
- I'm in perfect health.

- I live with a wonderful man.

January 8, 1991, a horrible rainy day, was probably the worst day of my life. With Michelle at my side, I went to see my oncologist, who by this time had all the data necessary to make a decision. I was still prepared for what I considered "the worst"...that is, he would tell me I had to have a mastectomy. Instead he said we would have to use chemo "to bring this tumor into an operable range." I was absolutely shocked. I said, "But the opposite of 'operable' is '*in*operable'!" He explained that this was *not* good news he was giving me. I asked him what the boundaries of the tumor were, and he told me they were what we felt. What he was telling me was that the *whole* breast constituted the possible outside definition of the cancer. This wasn't a tiny, definable lump, as before, but a raging cancer which could not be discerned easily on film or through other technologies.

I moved out toward the waiting room, and my knees buckled. Michelle came forward and held onto me. My next thought was that I would have to begin exactly the same regimen that I'd begun a year ago...the long drives out to Maryland to get the treatments. I went back into the examining room, where my doctor was sitting, slumped against the table, staring at his notes. I leaned against the door jam, asking him if I could get my chemo closer to home. His wife joined us, and they insisted that they be allowed to take care of me, not someone else. And so it would happen that way.

That evening I went to a birthday party for Michelle's husband, and I was not alone until I went to bed.

The next day I called Nancy in West Virginia to see how Nick was doing. This turned out to be a very valuable phone call. The fall before, Nick had had large malignant lumps all over his body; and after a few treatments with the same drugs I was about to use, his cancer had literally disappeared. I clung to this news, hoping that I could as easily find an answer for my own situation.

On January 17, I began an aggressive protocol designed for aggressive tumors...Novantrone, Vincristine, and Cytoxan. I was holding up fairly well until my doctor took out a ruler and, with his hand holding my breast, measured from one side to the other. I burst into tears. This was to be our tool to assess the progress we made…a simple gauge in inches.

On the way home I was so distressed that I *wanted* to pull over to the side of the road and get sick. I *wanted* to vomit, because I thought I could get rid of the terrible grief and anger I had accumulated. The irony was that I *couldn't* get sick. In fact, I made it through the series of treatments with virtually no side effects. In late January I went for a complete bone scan and a liver scan, both of which were fine. This, coupled with the good news about Nick, would see me through my tougher days.

I began to fall into a pattern of defining my life almost entirely by my medical situation. I was too consumed with the things I *couldn't* do, *couldn't* have, *couldn't* control. My acupuncturist had picked up on this and had cautioned me against continuing to filter everything through my medical problems.

About this time I returned to my support group, which now was a positive force. The women who had been steering the group toward self-pity and a recounting of old problems were no longer attending meetings. I also began to see that helping other women would be a part of my own recovery, so I became a very reliable member.

Another difficult facet of the treatment program was solved when Pattie gave me a key to her house and made a fresh bed for me to use after each visit to the doctor. This helped immensely. I had a prescription for a powerful tranquilizer, and I would drive the few miles to her house, take the pill, and fall into bed. She and I called this "going to La-la Land." She came and went while I slept; and the next day when my head was clear, I would go home. I'd never taken any mind-altering drugs, but I must say this really helped the anxiety and probably was one of the reasons I had no nausea.

By the second or third treatment we actually saw results. There was shrinkage in the breast, and it was moving freely against the chest wall. Then the rate of progress gradually slowed, and we began to talk mastectomy. The word didn't frighten me as much as I would have predicted, perhaps because I knew how bad a problem we were facing; and I was anxious to rid myself of this vile thing. I had my last chemo June 3, and I went for a mammogram three weeks later. Once again it was inconclusive.

I was trying to find ways to get outside myself, so I decided to do some volunteer work at Children's Hospital in D.C. This would turn out to be more than just a change in my lifestyle. It would teach me some valuable lessons about survival.

LEARNING COURAGE
by Helen Rash

This was not my first time working at Children's Hospital. In my late twenties I had been trained to be a volunteer at the old site on 13th Street in Washington, D.C. I had gone for a series of Saturday morning classes to learn about the various stages in a child's life and how hospitalization affects them at those times. As a part of our classes we had rotational assignments on several different wards to get us ready for the time when we would receive our permanent posts. I was able to handle my trial visits to the general hospital wards; but when the time came for me to try the burn ward, I didn't do well. They asked me to feed a little girl who had been burned over her entire body, and I found out later she died the next day. For a week or so I felt a kind of nausea when I thought about her. No volunteers were forced to accept an assignment to the burn ward, and I asked to be excused from any involvement with those children.

When in the summer of 1969 the classes were over, I was assigned for one evening a week to a floor where the patients were recovering from surgery or had been abused or neglected. I played with the children or, if they were very small, I held them or sang to them. There were times when a child had to go through treatment or tests with no family member present to comfort them. We were not allowed to become involved with the medical procedures, but sometimes we were asked to hold the child. I was very distressed by this...a child having to go through some awful phase of his life, even if for only a moment, without a parent to hold onto. Once a little girl about five was taken to the examining room so they could draw blood, and I went with her. They were having trouble finding a vein, so they had to smack the back of her hand to get one to rise. She screamed and cried. How could they explain that this was "for her own good"?

I learned too much about the children of the inner city and the dreadful things that can happen to them. One evening a little girl about eighteen months old was brought in and placed in one of the beds. When I moved to pick her up, the nurse told me not to. She said the baby had been systematically tormented by her parents, and she had a series of cigarette burns over her body as a result. The nurse explained that this child would not understand what I was doing if I picked her up and might even be more frightened than if left alone. I sat next to the bed and talked quietly to her. She was lying face down on the sheet, with her hand near her mouth. I put my arm on the sheet along-side hers, without really touching her. Eventually she took her hand and moved it up against my arm. She stayed like this for a while and then, very delicately, she lifted her baby finger, moved it, and tapped the back of my hand.

Sometimes the children who were brought in were almost beyond hope, like the little girl who'd spent her first four years lying in her crib staring up at the ceiling. She was so malnourished that she was retarded, and her body was flat down the back from being in that same position so long. Our task was to stimulate her by presenting new sounds, shapes, and colors for her to focus on. Some mothers had no money for milk, and when their babies cried, they gave them a bottle with water in it to suckle. These babies were slowly starving.

*   *   *   *

When I returned twenty-two years later to repeat the required training, the hospital had relocated to a beautiful new building in another part of D.C. Again we had to do rotational assignments on the various wards. Because of my recent experiences with IV chemotherapy, I was startled to see the children nonchalantly rolling their tall IV stands along with them to the playrooms. They had an amazing capacity for ignoring the metal "hat-rack" and the bags of fluid strung on them. The tiny children used the base and the wheels like a scooter and had me pull them along the halls on the way back and forth from their rooms to the play area. My blue smock was a sign that I was there for *only* fun. One little girl walked directly up to me and said, "You're a volunteer; you can't hurt me." And she turned on her heel and walked away.

One of my assignments was an evening on the cancer ward. The common areas were full of little pale bald children romping, coloring in books, cutting and pasting, and visiting with guests. I was to sit with a little girl named Cissie...about six years old. When I entered her room, she was huddled at the top of her bed on her pillow, hugging a stuffed animal. She was totally bald, and her ornate pink dress was the only evidence that she was a girl. I sat on the bed and talked to her; and like a little bird slowly hatching from its egg, she gradually straightened her legs, then her arms, and sat up. I'd brought a game with me, and eventually she became interested and was very excited. Her parents called; and after she'd talked for a few minutes, she said, "I have to go now. My volunteer is here." By the end of my stay, she was jumping up and down on the bed, flopping the IV tubing around as she waved her arms in the air.

An odd thing happened. When the time came for the volunteers to sign up for our permanent placements, the schedule went all the way around the table before I got to see it. By the time it reached me, there was very little left except the burn ward, so I decided to try it in spite of the memories left over from earlier days.

There were three levels of care on the burn ward: an isolation unit where the severely damaged children were cared for when they first arrived; a median level where only certain visitors were allowed and the children were still in critical condition; and a hallway which was basically like any other set of rooms in the hospital. My work was primarily on this latter corridor; however, I did spend some evenings in the mid-level area with a sweet young blond boy named Kenneth. He'd been so badly burned that he was wrapped in bandages almost entirely except for his face. This meant he was virtually immobilized.

In spite of his pain and a voice that was little more than a whisper, he wanted to play a board game. We spent long hours with the board on a bedside tray, with me tossing the dice for him and moving his marker the proper number of spaces. Sometimes he just signaled by rolling his eyes in the direction he wanted me to move the piece. There were times when the nurses had to come and take him to clean his wounds and change his dressings, and I saw the absolute horror in his eyes. I promised I would wait for him, and we would continue the game. We tacked a paper up on the wall, where we kept track of the number of games won and lost. He beat me. In the next few months I saw him move on to the regular hospital rooms, dressed like a typical child in tennis shoes and gown, able to walk the halls. This brought me a great deal of joy, and I took strength from his courage.

One evening I sat in the open hall area and held a little boy named Lamont whose face had been so badly burned that it was now totally pink. He was covered in some kind of ointment, and his face glistened. I helped him through supper, and then the nurse came to give him his bath. This upset him, so I promised that when he returned I would be sitting in the same chair, waiting to play. When he came back, he ran across the floor as if we'd known each other a long time, climbed up into my lap and hugged me tightly around the neck. He sat with his back to me, both of us facing the large table out in the hall where the children gathered to eat and play.

Eventually about six or seven members of his family came down the corridor and quietly sat in the chairs at the table with us. I was startled when he wrapped his feet back around my legs and pressed his body against my chest. He remained this way, totally silent. At first I felt awkward, since I would have expected him to climb down and head for whichever member of the group was his parent. Then I decided it was none of my business what happened there. I also realized that he might have had memories that somehow linked the fire and his family. He just said one thing, "My face itches." Then the woman who was the oldest of the relatives said softly, "Thank you for doing this." I told her I enjoyed being with the children, that Lamont in particular was very sweet, and that it was my pleasure to be able to help.

These weekly trips up into D.C. to be with the children continued for a number of months until a time when my life became more complicated, and I had to avoid being around sick people. When it ended, I missed it very much. I often felt that I had moved, as the children had, through several levels of pain, at first feeling very damaged, then hurt but starting to function, and at last, moving out into the world again.

WEEDING
by Helen Rash

Meantime, I was moving toward my mastectomy. I was absolutely convinced that I would go into the hospital, have the breast removed, be reconstructed, and walk out without a hitch. This thought was what sustained me. I met with my general surgeon, and he and my oncologist referred me to a plastic surgeon. The plastic surgeon seemed strangely subdued and told me I was a candidate for only *one* type of reconstruction...that which involved taking my own abdominal muscle, pulling it up to the chest area and building the breast with this muscle and a skin graft. By chance this was the option I was interested in anyway, so I didn't waiver in my intent. He said he needed to talk to the other members of my medical team and get back to me. That was a Thursday.

Four days later I got home late in the evening and found a message from his secretary on my machine, saying he wanted me to see another plastic surgeon for a second opinion. I had no way of talking this out with him that night, and I spent the rest of the evening in a very bad state of mind. I was terrified, not really understanding the true nature of my particular cancer and thus not recognizing the factors they were considering.

The next day I was able to get through to the first plastic surgeon. He told me he was recommending that we do the mastectomy, make sure the area was cancer free, then six months later go back and do the reconstruction. I didn't like what I heard, but it made sense. When I saw the second specialist, he told me the same thing. He also measured my abdomen and skin area and told me that, because I'd never been pregnant, my stomach muscles were tighter than someone who'd had children.

I decided I wanted to get on with the next step, so I immediately called my general surgeon and set up the mastectomy for Saturday, July 13, 1991. Because I'd had seven months to say the word "mastectomy" aloud, I was fairly calm about it, perhaps more so than most women who have to face this on very short notice and are still in a state of shock. My niece flew out to be with me, and she stayed at Pattie's house so she could be near the hospital.

Contrary to what one might expect, a mastectomy without reconstruction, when done by a skilled surgeon, is not particularly difficult physically for the patient. Within twenty-four hours, I was feeling well, strong, rested. I had very little difficulty with pain, nor was I frightened or depressed. Because I'd known about this vile tumor for so long, I was relieved to get it out of my body.

Once again I was told I had cancer in seven of the fifteen lymph nodes they'd removed from under the left arm. I kept telling myself that seven was better than fifteen out of fifteen. I'm always like the little boy in the well-known story…searching for the pony under the pile of manure.

On Monday they removed the surgical dressing, and I shed a few tears when I saw the long, clean incision on the left side of my chest. It was as if I were saying good-bye to an old friend. My surgeon came and sat with me…told me I could go home. He then said, "I want to tell you a story. It's just a story. Over fifteen years ago I did a mastectomy on a woman, and her prognosis was not good. A few years later she had a malignant skin lesion, which I removed. She's done fine ever since, so I asked her if she does anything special. She said, 'I meditate, and I take at least three grams of Vitamin C a day.'" I must add here that among the members of my medical team, all of whom respected each other, there was a complete range of opinions about non-traditional methods of healing. On one end was this surgeon, who believed in *all* possibilities: hypnosis, nutrition, Eastern approaches to healing, meditation, acupuncture. He encouraged me to try anything available. Of course, I was already one jump ahead of him in these areas, and no one had to convince me. At the other end of the spectrum was my oncologist, whose eyes would glaze over a little when I'd mention my forays into alternative forms of healing.

About this time I felt very detached from the world around me. It was as if my new body were a little boat in which I'd been set adrift. Even though there were lots of supportive people around, I really had not re-attached myself to my house, my job, my life in general. We keep in touch with the outside world through our physical bodies, our intellect, and our senses. All of these had been temporarily modified by my mastectomy. This sensation passed quickly, however.

Among my wonderful friends and family members I began to hear a subtle strain in their voices as they stood by and watched all that was happening, helpless to take any of the pain away.

On the first of August, I wrote in my diary about a dream I'd had. A man who owned a large aquarium decided to drain all the water and let the fish die. I ran around, trying to get drinking glasses filled with water, but I was able to save only a few of the fish.

SHOWER
by Jana Morgana

Standing in the shower
Soothing water
Feelings   My beautiful body
I have been hurt   Cut   Burned
Lumpectomy   Radiation
Breast so sensitive
I use soapy water
Squeezed drop by drop
Node sampling
Under arm   Numb   No feeling
Upper arm   Sharp   Shooting pains
Gently stroke from elbow to shoulder
Scared and gentle
Remember   I have had fine nerves cut
Large muscles and nerves
Stretched and traumatized
For my own good
To remove cancer and test for spread
My body and emotions
Have not gotten that message
With the cleansing water running over me
Sadness   Hurt   Flows out   Crying
My beautiful body

THE VIGILANCE MUST CONTINUE
by Lesley Tyson

the vigilance must continue
and the fear never truly recedes
after meeting every challenge
overcoming every obstacle
another small knot of tissue
waiting for the answer
which will tell me
how rough the road will be

WHOSE BODY IS THIS?
by Katherine Traynham

So one breast is way smaller than the other one. And it has a permanent tanned circle on one side from the radiation. The scar looks pretty good...the nipple is a little weird, but what the heck. I've started wearing "old lady" bras. The ones that look like armor. Need lots of support. Well, one breast does, at least...the other one just needs normal support.

It used to drive me crazy that I needed a bathing suit designed for a real person—the bottom was never right for the top. Now the right side of the top isn't right for the left side of the top. But there's still something there, so I can be grateful for that.

It just doesn't feel like me. It feels...thick. The sensation in the nipple is a little different, or is that my imagination? Funny, it used to be my favorite breast. Is that stupid? To have a favorite? For nursing. Or for sex, let's face it. It's not my favorite anymore. Or my husband's, I'll bet.

I'm not all that thrilled about the other one, either. It's sort of—flabby. Maybe the breast tissue is thinning out because of menopause (that's good—it will be easier to see a small cancer), or maybe it's because I gained so much weight and then lost some. Or maybe it's just that I'm forty-five and that's what happens, but I got distracted by cancer. I can't remember. I can't remember what it felt like when I was "normal" and I can't remember when it changed. I can't even decide if it is a change that's real or one I imagine because I'm crazed and nothing feels right anymore.

And another thing. My hands look like my mother's now. I should wear gloves when I garden or have my hands in water. They look like alligator skin and I don't use lotion enough. I think that fat freckle is an age spot starting. Of course, I've got all kinds of those little red dots that are a funny kind of freckle. The dermatologist says you get them after forty or so, when you stop making new, normal freckles. Great. They'll go well with my little purple tattoos. I can play dot-to-dot with a Magic Marker.

CAN YOU COME HERE WHERE I AM?

My fingernails don't look the same. God knows, my toe-nails don't. I thought I had a toenail fungus. It was just the chemo that "killed" them and now they're growing normally again. That'll take about a year. Everything's supposed to take a year: my blood work should be completely normal; I'll probably have back my regular hair instead of the baby-fine stuff that came in; my hair will "remember" that a bunch of it was gray; the residual arthritis in my joints should go away.

In a year, they'll know what's permanent and what was temporary—but will I look like myself again? Will I dance around the house to old rock and roll while I vacuum? Will I look at myself naked and not see a chubby, middle-aged woman? That's not because of breast cancer, that's just the calendar. But I didn't see it before. I don't like my toes, my belly, my teeth. It doesn't look like my fanny. It looks like the fanny of a woman who…has had cancer.

Is that it? I want to look the way I did before I had cancer. Nobody can tell much of a difference but me…but I *know*. And it looks different. I look older. Sadder. Puffy. I want to love my body again. I didn't love it at seventeen, or twenty-five. Or twenty-eight. I was actually pretty pleased with it from about thirty to thirty-eight. For eight out of my forty-five years, I loved my body. It did exactly what I wanted it to do. It felt solid. Responsive. Sexy. Mine.

I don't know whose body this is. It looks a lot like my mother's. She used to tell me she got a little shock every time she looked in a mirror, because inside she was still about thirty-two. Around age fifty or so, it started to be a real problem. She'd see her reflection and get a little jolt, "Omigosh! That's what I look like." But inside, it was the year she had me. She still looked great on the dance floor, inside.

She was always beautiful to me. I wish I were beautiful to me. I wish my breasts looked like they are mine. I don't care if they don't match, but I don't know whose they are.

CAUGHT OFFSIDE OFF GUARD
by Lesley Tyson

caught offside off guard
by the distorted reflection
out of the corner of my eye
the concave scarred mutilation
where my breast used to be
so evident in the sideways glance
this unbalanced deformity
scars hollows tattoos magnified
such a different reality
from facing myself head-on
where gentle survivor's eyes
see a strong beautiful woman
slightly wounded

NUDE BEACHES
by Rita Busch

I have had two mastectomies. Does that mean I can go swimming topless in public?

AS TIME PASSES
by Lesley Tyson

as time passes
it is almost
with a sense of surprise
that as i undress
i see the blank space and the scar
until that moment
there is no challenge
to my sense of wholeness and balance
even the evidence of my eyes
has little power
over my complete heart

CRYING

by Jana Morgana

Crying from not being good enough
Not doing it right   Punished
Holding it in   Why me
Stuffy   Swollen   Headache
Dark cloud
Crying I have done it
And I will do it again
Joyous   Miraculous   Alive
Free flowing clear mucus
Clear head and thinking
The world's mine
Exuberance   The sun is bright
Crying   Loved ones
Hurt   Leaving   Dead
I did the best I could
I have the connections forever
Crying   Illness   I am hurt
Wail   Shout
I feel the hurt   Body shaking
I am off balance and adjusting
I will regain myself   My life
I cry   I change   I heal

NOTES FROM A GARDENER
by Katherine Traynham

I don't know why it made me so furious, but it did. I have since found out the same stuff made lots of us angry. I was reading, reading everything I could get my hands on about cancer. Friends gave me books about self-healing, diet, meditation, music, attitude, positive imaging, everything. I soaked it up.

But I kept running across parts referring to a single study—the one where breast cancer comes on the heels of grief. All the new "experts" (or perhaps all the old experts had newly decided) there was evidence (studies, numbers, etc.) that an important loss, especially the loss of a mother or a child, looked like a precipitating factor in breast cancer. There was one whole evaluation just on daughters losing their mothers and how many of those daughters ended up with a breast cancer diagnosis within two years.

I was also reading that, based on how cells divide, my cancer, by the time I found it, was probably ten years old. When those wrongly-formed cells first divided, I was getting married again—not burying my mother. I was in a job I'd worked for all my life, making more money than ever, my daughter was starting second grade, and I was finally in love with a truly fine man.

I kept reading. It perhaps was the aggressive switch on the tumor that had reacted to the grief when my mother died of lung cancer. Eight months later, I found the lump in my right breast. The experts, no doubt, would nod sagely and talk about cancer going through slow and fast stages. Perhaps my grief had sent it into overdrive. It made me want to spit.

As I read, it seemed to me they were saying my love for my mother had tried to kill me. My desire to be involved with her treatment and illness for two years until her death had worn me down and signed my death warrant, too. What I read seemed to say to me that love was dangerous—but I believed it was terrible, powerful, and illuminating and the one thing we had to have or we really would die, one way or another. It made no sense to me that God had set up Nature so that the more important someone

Can You Come Here Where I Am?

was to you, the more likely losing them would make cancer cells grow.

It was a stupid, simplistic connection, but it's the one I made when I read what the "experts" said. I thought they meant that if we didn't love so deeply, so terribly, we would never make breast cancer cells when we grieved.

Even if it were true, I wanted to know—so what? Why tell us? What were we supposed to do? Bury our dead and not grieve? Try not to love so deeply, so that when we lost that love, we wouldn't self-destruct? It made me crazy with rage. It made no sense. I could understand the grief killing you if you lost a child—what an unnatural, awful sacrifice! But parents? It's the natural order of things. We've been doing it for millions of years. We bury our mothers and fathers. How could Nature be set up to take us out for its own ordered system? And if I couldn't trust Nature with that, how could I trust Nature to help me fight cancer??? Hmmmm?

I felt I was left with only two choices: Love this much, even if it kills you, or: Don't love so much and miss the important stuff.

I didn't like either. I invented another paradigm I like better.

It's apparently a lot like spending a lot of time in your garden. If an intruder comes and ransacks your house while you're in the garden, you can hardly know it's happening, can you? When you aren't in the garden, you can manage the house and turn things on and off and keep it straight and pick up and dust. When you're in the garden, you let the house go for awhile, because you need to be out in the garden!

Some people live their whole lives in the house. They arrange their days around the interior. They hardly get out of themselves, but they have an orderly dwelling. Spotless, maybe. Other people, like me, love the garden. The house can fall apart, but I'm out in the garden with the flowers and bulbs and dirt and it feels wonderful. Maybe the house doesn't look so good, but it doesn't fall apart...unless an intruder comes. I may have been a disinterested housekeeper, but I wasn't careless or irresponsible. I was just busy in the garden.

There was a burglary while I was busy in the garden. A break-in. Some things were damaged. If I want, I can lock myself in the house and spend the rest of my life guarding it. I'll have a spotless, fortress-like house and unless they come back with guns, I'll be fine.

But then I'd never get back out to the garden.

Maybe you just can't be two places at once.

I'm not so furious anymore with what I read about grief and breast cancer. I'm not leaving the neighborhood because of one break-in.

Frankly, the only reason I have the house is for its garden, anyway.

DREAM DREAM DREAM
by Daena Kluegel

Since surgery I have had a recurring nightmare. I am involved in something which demands my attention. I am so very busy, but suddenly I brush my hands together and something is missing. I look down and my diamond engagement and wedding rings are missing. I become frantic, looking for the rings everywhere. Where are they? I run desperately up and down stairs and in and out of rooms searching for the rings. I ask everyone I meet to help me: my daughter, my friends, my son, my husband, but they all are too busy working on household chores. Usually I wake at this point and must reassure myself by finding those rings still on my hand. Pretty Freudian?

Then, there is my repeated dream of having tea with HRH the Queen of England, in a splendid setting out of doors with woods nearby. The Queen is dressed in regal formality and I am equally formal in attire with heels, lovely dress, and gloves. As we sit chatting on our cushioned white chairs, I balance my bone china tea cup delicately and smile. Then, her pet deer wanders by and I reach out to touch its antlers. The antlers dislodge! They remain in my hand and the deer disappears. I try to hide the antlers behind my back and be nonchalant while making witty and brilliant conversation and hoping that She doesn't notice! Meanwhile, other people enter the area: servants, nobles and uniformed footmen. I become more and more anxious that I will be discovered with the antlers in my hands and that no one will believe my explanation of the accident. Another voyage into Freudian metaphors.

It has been seven years and the frequency of the dreams has lessened but not the intensity. I wonder whether this is mental scar tissue which will never disappear but will fade with time?

DREAM A LITTLE DREAM
by Katherine Traynham

I didn't have any trouble sleeping. I was scared to death for several weeks during every waking moment. Obsessed. Had to get on with it, know everything, start treatment *now*. Get it over with *now*. But when I'd lie down, I'd be asleep in seconds. Sleep was always my favorite escape. I sleep through terrible storms. I slept constantly when my daughter's father and I separated. It's how I cope. Or escape. Same thing. To me, anyway.

And even though I'm a night person, I can sleep when I'm stressed. I'll stay up if there's something I want to do, but I won't stay up just to worry. I'll go to sleep instead.

And I didn't have nightmares. People asked me, "Are you having trouble sleeping?" Heck, no. The doctors would ask, "Are you sleeping okay? Any nightmares?" Nary a one. I wasn't being chased in the dark. I wasn't falling down an endless hole. None of the classics.

After about a month, I began to dream. It was the one I did in visualization. I dreamed I was on "our" favorite beach—mine and my husband's. Where we go every year. (Where we've made love, sneaking, in the dark, on a sandy towel, with the waves whooshing.) I dreamed it was day and we were dancing. (He doesn't dance. That's how I knew it was a dream.) I was whole and happy and graceful and thin—no, not just thin. Supple. Slinky. I wore a beautiful, sheer summer dress—maybe voile. It floated on the breeze, but my movements were more graceful than even that dress. My husband was smiling at me the whole time. He held me in his arms and we laughed and danced all over that beach. I was barefoot and on tiptoes. I swirled and leaned away and turned under his arm and we were all alone in the sun and the breeze and the waves tried to catch our feet as we danced near the water.

I dreamed it over and over and over. In the daytime, I'd listen to meditative music and dream it awake. At night, I'd dream it in Technicolor. It was better than any movie I've ever seen. It was in the future and we were together, dancing not for joy, but for happiness, surely. I would look forward to going to sleep because I knew I would probably dream that dream. I loved it because it was just us. Because we were fascinated with each other. Because it was graceful, whether we are or not. Because I looked timeless—not that much younger than I really am, but not as old as I feel. Because we were whole and healthy and crazy about each other and uninterested in anything except each other and the dancing. I feel wonderful describing it. I dream it still and can almost decide to dream it when I go to bed at night.

It is an icon for me. A visual mantra. A focal point. I've had some pretty crazy dreams in my life, but none of them felt important, the way this one does. Is it us, or the dress, or the dancing? Is it the beach? This beach is where I first felt deep happiness. Not the exhilarating joy of having a baby, or the celebratory shout of an achievement, or the quiet pleasure of a satisfied life. Deep, deep happiness. We rarely danced, but we did on occasion and just after we fell in love, we went to this beach for the first of many times. I had never been so whole-heartedly turned toward another human being before. And on that beach, I loved a man and watched the porpoises play a hundred yards offshore. I don't even swim, but I could have joined them that day.

I will dream this dream, in deliberate measure, until I can dance it in the sun, awake. It will be a marker for me that the cancer is a footnote, not the title of my life. Maybe that's the great attraction in this dream. There is no doctor, no machine, no importance for my breasts, no attention to scars, physical or psychic, no blood work, no charts, no hospital nearby. My husband doesn't look at me with care or concern—he just looks at me because I am his. The cancer is neither here nor gone—it isn't "before cancer" in this dream, it just doesn't matter that it is after. In this dream, I am a woman with the man I love, on a beach, in the sun, dancing barefoot on my tiptoes in a flowing dress, and the whoosh of the waves makes the music we dance to and the sea gulls whirl in lazy circles, curious above us and the porpoises mimic our minuet just off the shore in the water where it begins to turn green not blue and the sand crabs dodge us as they dart in the whitest sand in my favorite place in the universe. And I will dream this dream until I dance it in the sun and there is no cancer in the world that will keep me from it.

THE COLLECTOR
by Katherine Traynham

I'm saving up.
I'm saving books.
I'm saving things for someone who's not here yet.
I'm writing letters to people not on this earth.
They're yet to be.
I've culled the photographs.
I've named the faces on the back.
I've packed the boxes with the baby clothes.
I made the list.
Of who made what.
What Grandma knitted
For my baby when she was a baby.
There are tags.
I put them there.
Of what I made and in what year—
It's all right there!
The Easter outfit
Complete with hat
The set of Peter Rabbit dishes,
Crewelled lambs from my sister.
Then the dolls—
Both mine and hers.
The one my sister gave.
The one from Mom.
It's all for one.
This only child of mine.
And then she said the magic words.
"What if you don't..."
"What if you aren't..."
"If I have a little girl..."
"When I grow up..."
And then I knew.
I wasn't through.
I had my life arranged for anyone to see.

For her to find me (just in case I'm gone).
To find our smiles, this mother
And the ones before.
Eight generations
Six silver spoons,
Milk pitcher, teapot,
Diamond ring and amber beads.
I lined us up.
The things we gave
In perfect order so its meaning could be found.
But she was wanting one more thing from me.
A thing that would go on into the future.
If I didn't.
If I couldn't.
Not from me to her or them to her
Through me.
And so I bought a doll for no one yet.
Not for my daughter or my sister or for me.
For someone
Not here.
Not yet.
A someone to be someday to me.
Grandchild.
Granddaughter.
Spectacular doll.
A porcelain face
A head that turns
In a satin dress—
A ball gown in red,
With beads down the front,
And shoes made of suede,
And a cascade of dark hair.
Like my mother's.
Like my daughter's.
And full lips and eyelashes that curl.

And I packed her away, in the boxes of me.

144

With the things that were mine
And the lists that are signs.
And she's cradled in tissue.
Has a tag with her name.
I have hopes that I'll place her
In some chubby sweet arms.
Someday.
I'm saving up.
I'm packing away.
The books and the letters.
I'm writing the lists.
It's all in the boxes.
So I can be found someday.
Just in case I'm not here to tell you.

STUPID PEOPLE TRICKS
by Helen Rash

For years I went to the same radiology clinic for my mammograms, and each time I had the same technician. She was a heavy-set, plain woman who went about her business efficiently. As my medical history grew, it became harder and harder for me to fit all my surgeries, radiation treatments, and chemotherapies into the few lines devoted to these on the clinic form. When I had only one breast remaining and needed to have a follow-up image to see how I was doing, I did my best to complete the paperwork. I was sitting in her area, wearing my little paper cape, when she came in carrying my form. She stood over me, grasping the paper in both hands. She said, "This isn't right. We're either going to fill this out correctly, or we're not doing it at all." She then tore the paper up in front of me. I was stunned that she could be so severe, especially given what was in my background. But I was even more stunned when my letter of complaint about the incident was later shared with her, so she knew who had lodged the complaint! The doctor in charge had obviously told her, since the technician wrote me a bizarre letter, saying her "true supervisor" was God.

* * * *

When I first developed cancer in my liver, I was very jaundiced. I decided one day to drop by a French cafe for a light lunch. As I took my tray and began my walk through the food line, a young Frenchman behind the counter asked, "Excuse me, Miss. Eez eet zee *livaire?*" I knew immediately he was talking about my obvious yellow color. I said yes, it was my liver. Then I moved on to the next stop, the soups. He followed. "Do you mind if I ask you what the disease eez?" I replied that it was cancer. He said he'd attended medical school. (If anyone ever again says to me in a restaurant "Is it the liver?" I'll probably say, "No, I'm going to have the quiche.")

THIS MOMENT
by Jana Morgana

Every Moment I prepare for Dying
This is from Being
Smothered   Shaken   Choked
Which is it
Adult abusers did Not Kill Me
Or   I chose to live
At this moment   Do I choose to Live
After Breast Cancer
I am coming out of
Expecting to Die
I am using all that has happened
To Live Now

ZERO TOLERANCE
by Katherine Traynham

Who the heck am I anyway? That is, who am I, *after cancer?*
I've been waiting for the big change—the making of me into a
better person—wiser, more giving—a sort of saintly version of
myself, because something bad happened to me.

It's not happening. I don't know if I'm worse, but I'm certainly not better. It's not as if I'd sat around the house for years
eating bonbons, unconcerned with the fates of those around me.

I'd been a decent daughter, worked in television for fifteen
years, achieved some modest success by arriving at network just
before my thirty-second birthday. I'd quit all that when I'd re-
married, to be at home with children. We'd taken in a foster son.
I participated moderately at church, where I felt I might have some
talents, and sometimes just where others thought I had a talent.

I wasn't out saving the world—and I'm still not. I wrote a
weekly newspaper column with a good friend, and we'd been
doing this for six years—we kept writing all through my cancer
treatment, though no doubt she sometimes carried my load of it.
We wrote about my cancer twice in a year, otherwise something
less self-centered.

I keep looking for the changes—am I better? Did walking
through this fire make me a better, kinder, gentler Kathe? Nope.
I am either unteachable, or I don't see the changes. If anything,
I'm a less gentle version of the cancerless Kathe.

I want what I want now. I want it my way. I want time to do
what I want. I want people to shut up and snap out of it. I am
impatient for people to get busy doing good, fun things—they
don't have to be meaningful. Just less bitching, please. Less criti-
cizing, for pity's sake. Less moving around of the furniture and
more sitting on it.

I don't mind if people don't believe what I believe. I am not
insulted that they have a different faith, a different view, a different—life. This one is mine, this is how it looks to me, this is
what I believe, this is how I work the puzzle given to me. They
don't have to do theirs my way. They can even question how
I'm doing mine—I'll listen.

I want people to love one another. Isn't that silly and cheap and juvenile? I just want the bickering, the hatred, the unflattering comparisons to stop. I want people to get over being angry about past injustices and crap nobody can change in their lives. If their mothers were awful I want them to shut up and live on, the best they can.

If men are creeps, then toss one out and do without, but nobody does, of course. If having children is such a burden, then by all means, don't have them on my account.

There are so many pointless struggles, I think. Where will we get the strength for a real battle if we're so busy straining against all this meaningless crap that doesn't have to be a struggle?

I have a couple of friends who are depressed. One of them seems to be enjoying it, and I feel cruel when I say that. I don't know what's wrong with him. I'm just tired of hearing about it. He's got the same problems at forty that he had at twenty. And he's doing the same thing about it—nothing.

Here's how I'm different: my sympathy filter got replaced. The new one is working only for people who do the best they can and don't enjoy the bad parts. The new me doesn't even feel sorry for me. The new me wants to stop wasting time. How many hours do I have in this life? How many of them am I going to spend listening to people complain about their kid's soccer coach? I can tell you right now: zero.

SWIM FOR YOUR LIFE
by Daena Kluegel

My surgeon wanted me to exercise and he thought my habit
of swimming half a mile several times a week would help me
regain flexibility. He thought three weeks was soon enough to
start swimming. I waited for six weeks as I was having trouble
just doing the Reach to Recovery exercises for the first three
weeks. There was the added problem that I was a psychological
coward about what I'd look like in swimwear. I had started the
treatments to expand my skin for a silicone implant, but I still
was scarred and flat and felt conspicuous. I was not about to go
out and buy a new mastectomy suit *and* prosthesis (falsie, as I
called it). I finally got bored and miserable enough to make the
attempt. My dear friend Mary Beth sensed my fears and declared
she really needed some exercise. Would I go to the local high
school pool with her for a swim? I agreed warily. Once inside
the building, I quickly hung up my street clothes under which I
had worn my suit, and rushed into the water. Safe in the shim-
mering, glistening liquid of the pool, I started to swim the breast
stroke. I was so stiff but I made a valiant effort for six circuits of
the twenty-five-yard lane. Instead of getting faster as I usually
did, I got slower and slower. I guess Mary Beth noticed, as she
said that she was so out of shape and had to quit, (she was an
aerobic instructor). We headed for the showers which were all
open. I decided that it was now or never for me, so I peeled off
the wet suit, took a deep breath and walked briskly into the
shower area. I felt as if everyone was aware of my scars, my lack
of symmetry where my breast should be. I was toweling dry when
I noticed a knot of teenagers at the far end of the dressing room.
They were all giggling, so I convinced myself they were laughing about and staring at me, although, without my glasses, I
certainly couldn't be sure what anyone was looking at or even
looked like. My throat constricted and my eyes started to smart.
How dare they? I straightened my shoulders and dressed holding
an imaginary conversation with those gaping girls. As we left
the steamy locker room and went out into the cold March air, I

felt stronger. I felt hopeful that I could return to a more normal routine now that I had faced down the dreaded first time.

I love swimming. It is warm and relaxing in the water like reclining in a wet, loving womb, a quiet world of blues and greens. Swimming stretches my muscles and mind as I get a chance to think during the rhythm of the strokes and turns. I often find I have worked out a problem or become inspired during my swim. When I am angry or frustrated, I can slap the water as hard as possible and defuse the anger. I leave the pool invigorated and strengthened. I remember how close I came to giving up my solace and letting the disease take even more from my life than it already had.

ISO

by Helen Rash

After my lumpectomy and all my treatments were done, I flew to Illinois to see my family. By chance on the plane I sat next to a young woman who was from the Midwest and who'd changed her lifestyle in order to fulfill her primary goal: to be happily married and raise a family. She'd worked for a high-powered law firm and had taken a drastic cut in pay to work for the government so she'd have more free time. We began talking about how hard it was to meet really decent men with the values we prized...and she mentioned she'd had good luck with personal ads.

This planted an idea in my mind; and a few weeks later, while vacationing at the beach, I drafted an ad. It began "Energetic, sophisticated redhead..." and went on to say that I had traditional values and was looking for a man who also placed a high value on friends and family. I put the ad in the *Washingtonian* "In Search Of" column and also answered nine ads from men in my general age range.

I went into this with an open mind, figuring I would probably have the same general level of success as I would with any segment of the male population. During the early fall I had a lot of what I called "Coke dates" with the people who'd answered my ad, or, more typically, whose ads I'd answered. These were always in public places...bars and restaurants...and I drove my own car so I'd be safe and free to leave at will. I spent so much time one week doing this that I jokingly told my friends that I was beginning to feel like a high-class call girl.

Had I judged the whole experience by the first meeting I had with one of these men, I probably would have thrown in the towel immediately. I responded to his ad, and he called me so we could talk. We then made arrangements to meet at a Vie-de-France Café at a big shopping center. He was going on afterwards to a picnic. When I first met him, I was startled, because he was dressed in rumpled clothes which probably were in need of washing, judging from the slight odor which seemed to follow him as he got in line to get his drink. During the whole conversation he disputed almost every issue that came up. As a result, it was difficult to just relax and have a nice chat. The thing that bothered me the most, however, was that I had written a letter describing my background and the kinds of things I enjoyed; and he never bothered to show any interest in any of it. I'd just assumed that someone with even the slightest social skill would pick up on that as a way of reaching out to the person sitting across the table. All in all, it was a real waste of time, but I didn't let this discourage me from going ahead with other men.

Some of the ads were very creative. One group of twelve businessmen said they were looking for twelve women to invite to a cocktail party. The women were supposed to write something that would get them an invitation. I relied almost entirely on the fact that I was a redhead, and how many redheads did they have on their list? I wound up going.

I kept all the letters and things in a shoe box, and my friends began referring to the men as "The Shoe Box Guys." I actually had several ongoing relationships as a result of all this, and it was good to get back to socializing. The men were all polite and decent to me, but I didn't find anyone who really suited my needs.

In the spring of 1992, I tried again, this time after my mastectomy. I answered four ads. One man called me and, with my letter in hand, talked about all we had in common: both from farming towns in Illinois; both of us went to the University of Illinois at the same time; both of us liked a broad spectrum in music, and so on. He had a husky, relaxed Midwestern voice, what I call an "astronaut's voice." I immediately had a sense of trust about him. I felt, given my vulnerability, that I should avoid lounge lizards and anyone else who would leave me feeling more insecure than I had been before.

We had dinner together, and I was very comfortable. He was tall, lanky, athletic. Not a good-looking man, but an attractive man. If I were casting a movie I'd probably choose a Sam Shepherd type to play his role. We went on to start dating. He did not come on to me sexually at first, and I was pleased about that. I knew, because I was wearing a prosthesis, that I would have to tell him fairly soon about the surgery. I also knew that the timing would have to be intuitive, since there's no easy way to get into the subject. One night we were eating supper at a restaurant, and we began to discuss self-healing through nutrition and vitamins. When I listed all the vitamins I was on, he asked why all the antioxidants? I could feel this would be a good time to tell him. So I did. He expressed real concern.

He then said, "Did I tell you about my daughter?" Since I knew he had one in college, I asked if he meant that child. He said no, the one who had died of cancer. I know I showed concern and continued to sit upright in my chair, but emotionally I just liquified and slid onto the floor. I knew that the death of a young child is an event that some people never put behind them, and I also could see how this could affect my time with him.

In spite of all this, we continued to see each other. I bought some pretty teddies and hid them in the bathroom cupboard, thinking that some time we might wind up in bed. When we first made love I had no left breast, and I had just returned to radiation; so I had a large green circle drawn on my chest. This didn't seem to bother him. He was a gentle and generous lover, and I was very glad that my first experience with my new body was going so well.

What finally ended the relationship was the specter of his daughter. He was filled with grief, even after ten years, and he couldn't seem to look at me without remembering. He told me one time my hair was the same color as hers. About six months later we tried again, but it just didn't seem to work. He was always tenderhearted and honest; so I didn't feel wounded or at fault for the failure of the friendship. I *was* grateful for the chance to try to be seductive and normal with someone who could deal with that part of me.

YOUR TOUCH
by Lesley Tyson

your touch carries me
beyond myself
i can almost believe
you don't notice
my missing breast
as you reach for me
again

KUDOS TO ...
by Katherine Traynham

My best friend who came immediately when I said, "It's malignant."

The friends who prayed (out loud) for me and risked it all.

My stepdaughter who cried and let me know she loved me.

The nurse who put her phone number in my hand, just as I woke up, and said, "I had positive nodes—eight years ago. Call me anytime."

The surgeon who sat down while I cried and said, "I know this is hell. Listen to me."

The radiologist who called to apologize for someone else's rudeness.

My sister for saying "I love you" before we hang up the phone.

My father, whose last note to me came with roses and said, "With all my heart, I love you."

The women in my Bible study group who don't kick me out, no matter what I say I believe.

My husband, for remembering the exact date that I found the lump in my breast.

The friend who brought cookies in a basket.

The one who sent flowers.

The anesthesiologist who couldn't hit a vein and offered to buy me a drink, instead.

The female doctor, when I said, "It always comes back, doesn't it?" who looked in my eyes and said, "Who told you that? He's a liar."

My daughter, for still bringing me her problems, because I'm still strong enough to handle them.

The friend who had just buried his wife because of cancer but insisted he wanted to know all about mine.

All the women who told me, "I had breast cancer, too."

The friend who had it ten years ago, who led me through the first (and worst) tunnels.

My doctor's receptionist who, while losing her sister, cheered for me, living.

The surgeon's wife, because she held my hand.

My husband, for making love to me like it was ten years ago.

The friend whose child had bone cancer but acted as if mine was important, too.

The woman in the waiting room who was always happy to see me again.

The woman I don't know who hugged me and cried the day we both finished radiation.

All the women with breasts and all the ones without them, and everyone who loves them.

RANDOM ACTS OF KINDNESS
by Daena Kluegel

How do you thank all of those people who helped you through the turmoil of diagnosis and treatment? I'm referring to the acquaintances who went out of their way to call or send funny cards. The teachers that I worked with took a collection of cheery, funny, and downright irreverent items in a huge basket to my house with instructions to read one per day during treatment. One teacher dropped off a batch of still-steamy muffins at my house on the way (it really was out of her way) to her job at a school across the county. Prayer chains were alerted of my need, even a Muslim prayer group. Meals appeared regularly at our home. There were friends who scoured the library for information. Young women used their computer data bases for the latest information about breast cancer treatment and brought it to me as soon as they left work. I never lacked for entertainment, friends brought tapes of books, videos of Lucy or Fawlty Towers and old, old movie classics.

Two exceptionally faithful and compassionate friends took turns bringing me to my chemo treatments. They planned a treat after every treatment such as a visit to an art gallery or lunch or a movie every time, so I might be nauseated, but I was never bored! They seemed to have nothing else that had to be done on those days, and they are both very busy women. They also helped to plan and orchestrate a "Survivor" party which I gave for myself after all the treatment and reconstruction was finished.

The Montessori teachers gathered at my house the night before my first chemo treatment. We were rowdy and hilarious. We were interrupted by my Mormon neighbor who wanted to give me a "Blessing." I tried to accept it in good grace until he said that I would not have needed surgery or chemotherapy if I had enough faith. I did not want to insult him but had to set him straight, and I think I was more restrained than is usual for me. I just said that I never felt I could require God to heal me in any specific way. I would accept any way in which it came to be accomplished, whether by a skillful medical doctor or a miracle. Did that put a damper on the evening? Not a bit! We continued far into the evening to laugh and act silly, which certainly helped fit me for the stress of chemo. Surely, laughter is the best medicine!

I am reminded of a story told by a fellow survivor. In the midst of her treatment, she was frantically concentrating on returning every dish which was brought full of family meals, to the owner filled with fresh cookies or such. Finally, a seventy-five-year-old neighbor said to her, "You just don't get it, do you? It's not 'pay it back,' but 'pass it on!'" I hope I can continue to remember to pass it on, until one day there is no more need because we will have beaten breast cancer as we did the polio epidemic of my youth.

CANCER? WHAT A HOOT!
by Katherine Traynham

Even serious stuff can be funny. Have you heard this one?

"So, my mother, who knew she would soon die of cancer, made me go with her to pick out her casket and dress because she figured my father couldn't take it. She was a real classic dresser. Suits. Low-heeled pumps. The tailored look.

"To my surprise, she chose a lavender dress with frills. It looked like something Blanche would wear in *A Streetcar Named Desire*. Real fading Southern Belle stuff. Then she chose the most elaborate casket in the whole place. A grayish-mauve model with flounces around the pillow and lining and white china medallions with hand-painted flowers at every joint and corner. It was the least like her of anything I've ever seen.

"'How do you like this color?' she wanted to know. 'Fine.' 'Do you think it will make me look jaundiced?' 'It's fine, Mother.' I wanted out of this.

"'Tell me the truth, do you think the dress will go okay with the lining?'

"I couldn't stand anymore. 'Truthfully, Mom, I don't think there is a casket in the world they could put you in where I'd look at you in it and think, gee, she looks great in there!'

"Mom patted my hand understandingly. 'Honey, I'm not trying to look great,' she explained. 'I just don't want to look like a corpse!'"

Or this one:

"'I hope my hair has time to grow back in before I die,' a woman told her friend.

'Well, maybe it will,' the friend said, 'but you've always got your wig.'

"'I know, I just hate to be buried in a wig instead of my own hair.'

"'Katherine,' the friend chided, 'I've known you for thirty years and I had no idea you were so vain!'

"'It's not vanity. I don't care what I look like,' the woman smiled. 'Wigs are just so hot!'"

Or this one:

"One day my friend Nancy called me. 'Let's go shopping!' she said. Nancy had finished radiation and was about to start chemo. She never wanted to spend money, so I got dressed in a hurry.

"'What's the big occasion?' I wanted to know.

"'I've lost so much weight, it's the first time I've been a size eight since I was in college. I'm going to buy everything in the store,' she laughed.

"'Yeah, but you're so cheap,' I teased. 'You never want to spend any money on yourself.'

"'That's the best part! I'm going to get a whole new wardrobe, and if I don't make it, my husband will have to pay off Visa himself!'"

WHERE THE RUBBER MEETS THE ROAD
by Katherine Traynham

Here are the things I had to figure out because I had cancer:

Who I am, What I'm going to do about cancer, How much I want to live, What's really important, Who do I really, really love, Who really, really loves me, and What happens now.

Here are the things I had already figured out before I had cancer:

Why is this happening, Why is it happening to me, Is there a God who cares, and What happens when I die.

The things my mother taught me as a child about faith and forever still hold. In youth, I questioned everything and examined all I could about what others believed. And I came to my faith in my head as well as in my history. You never know how good it works until it has to work in both life and death. My mother's faith was simple. She didn't complicate things with rules. Here is what I came to know her faith to be:

God is love. Love breeds love. Love responds to love. Love makes no distinctions. Love pushed away dies. Don't push God away. The rules aren't to keep you from having fun, they're to keep you from getting hurt. Forgive everything. Trust Love.

She believed, and I believe, that we will be with God someday, after death, more surely than we can be "with" Him now. She believed, and I believe, that He loves us more than we can understand love. That He would never allow my daughter to survive and yours to starve to death. Or choose some to be stricken and others to escape. It is simply what happens in a world with its own rules and laws that allow us to be free of Him, if we wish.

And so, there is no "why me?" for cancer unless there is a "why me?" for food and the United States, and a warm house, and freedom. There is no "specialness" conferred that exempts us from life. He loves me, and if a human parent would pace the floor and cry that I am stricken, so would He. Within His natural laws, He will use everything possible to do for me what Love does for Beloved.

Several years before I got cancer, our pastor told a group of us that prayer might be more to get us in line with God than to get God to do what we want. More to open us up to doing for others in need, than to get God to do what we want for those in need. I raised my hand. "I understand what you're saying, but if it's all the same to you," I said, "if I ever get cancer, please pray that I'll be healed. I don't know how God works and just in case, pray not only that I'll be comforted, and that you'll know what to do for me, but that I will be miraculously and completely healed. Just in case that's how He works." And we laughed.

And when I got cancer, a deeply spiritual friend remembered. She said, "We are coming to pray for you, because of what you said." And ten women (and one of their sons) came to pray for me, for healing, for God's Love, for miracles, for smart doctors and effective treatment, for comfort, for wisdom. And it was the first time I felt there was a healing place for me in the hearts of my friends.

Some say you can only be healed with great faith. That if you waver even a little, the formula is not right. That would be as if my daughter came to me, injured, and until she said the magic words, I would not bandage her wounds. Doesn't sound like love to me.

Some say God heals or doesn't arbitrarily and we don't understand it. That would be as if I had two children, both injured, and I bandaged one but not the other, without explanation. Doesn't sound like love to me.

Some say death is a healing. God can let one thing kill you to keep you from suffering something worse later, and you just don't know what's coming, but He does. In the middle of chemo, I saw my internist. He said, "You're going to do fine. This is going to take care of the cancer, and you'll live a long, long time." "And then," I teased, "I'll get some other horrible disease and die from that?" "Yes," he laughed. "My goal is for you to live long enough to die of something else!"

Some say God has a plan. That He has it all mapped out, and when we take a wrong turn somewhere, we throw everything off kilter. We've missed the plan. Here is the food that and when we take a wrong turn somewhere, we throw everything off kilter. We've missed the plan. Here is the food that feeds the heart of my faith: God is love. He laughs with me, mourns with me, suffers with me, celebrates with me, is with me. And will be. And I will be with Him. I may be deeply disappointed, but I will not be discarded. If I can love my children so deeply, so completely, so desperately, and I am so selfish, this God can love me deeply, completely, desperately, perfectly. I can sometimes find His presence here. I will surely be taken to that Presence when I die. And the rules, or the plan, or the healing, or the disappointment, is nothing to the Love.

For some, this is not enough. For me it is more than I ever expected or deserved.

NEW BABIES
by Katherine Traynham

Thank you so much for having a baby. Thank you for calling me, inviting me to the shower, including me in all your plans. I am so thrilled to be involved in something that's about living and starting and wondering and planning and trusting. I can't think of anything more wonderful right now.

A neighbor thought it was too sad. Said she didn't know how I could be expected to celebrate, with all the funerals this year. All the doctors. All the sickness. People should be more considerate, she said. She thinks people shouldn't tell me when their biopsies come back clear. That I might feel sad that mine didn't.

She must be nuts. I love it every time somebody gets a good report. I don't feel a bit jealous that it's not me. Everybody who lives, who struggles on, who keeps going, who has a baby, who starts a new job, who runs a marathon, is doing me a huge favor by telling me about it.

I am so tired of doctors and tests and symptoms and side-effects. I'm so tired of my every thought being about me. I can hardly wait for someone else to tell me how they're doing.

I was so grateful when a dear friend asked me to be her child's godparent—in the middle of my chemo! I draped a scarf over my head, parked a hat on top, dressed in my best suit, and held that baby while he was christened. I was so happy to do it. So happy to be included. So thrilled to still be in the middle of living.

Thank you for having babies. For putting them in my arms. For sending me the announcements. For expecting me to celebrate. You can't protect me from the bad things in life. For God's sake, please don't try to protect me from the wonderful.

THANK GOD, MY CLOSETS AND DRAWERS ARE A MESS
by Daena Kluegel

When I was recovering from surgery and having chemo-therapy treatments, one of the strategies which I used to give myself the illusion of maintaining control was to set goals for each day. It was usually some small and easily accomplished task. One that could be seen as completed fully each day. Thus, I felt that I was making a difference and not being completely useless, an unprofitable fungus upon the healthy body of the family. Some of these tasks were to finish putting all my collection of photos into photo albums, a welcome labor as most photos are taken of happy times which are fun to remember and this lifted my spirits to recall those times. Another task was to clean out and rearrange all those drawers in various bureaus, dressers and desks throughout the house. I felt very virtuous and proud to look at what I had wrought each day, because I was still in charge. In spite of a twice-a-week household helper, family, and friends cooking and running errands, I was doing something which needed doing.

When my daughter was diagnosed and underwent her sur-gery and chemotherapy and radiation treatments, I turned again to my sanity saver. I cleaned all the closets, but then I discov-ered that I had a driving need at all hours of day and night to clean my basement. I felt especially driven when Beth's treat-ments were most harsh and difficult or we were awaiting test results. I spent countless hours and energy upon this. I threw out old love letters from boyfriends I could no longer remember and who are probably living under bridges somewhere. Of course, I read every one of them. I wondered why I had kept them? What was my need to carry them with me in every move we made from house to house all these years?

It was very therapeutic. I felt I was cutting out calluses and old, dead tissue. I gave hundreds of books away. I made a clean sweep of memorabilia from high school and college. Everything was orderly and clean. Once again, I felt I had managed to grasp some control in an out-of-control situation.

In the play, *Mama's Bank Account*, Mama comes home from the hospital after her child has had an appendectomy and prepares to scrub the floor. The family chides her, reminding her that she only did this the day before. She says that she knows that, but sometimes you just have to get down on your knees. To that I would add that when you do not know what to do and are completely miserable, why not do something that you'd never do when you were not miserable?

That all happened over five years ago, and today I am so busy, I hardly notice my drawers. I quickly close the doors to the closets lest they, like Fibber McGee's legendary closets, explode outward over the room. I am delighted to say that my housekeeping is pretty hit-or-miss. Thank God my drawers and closets are a terrible mess!

LIGHTEN THE LOAD
by Helen Rash

Because I have lymphedema in my arm, I'm not supposed to lift heavy things. I told my brother that when I get home from the grocery store, I leave the nonperishables in the trunk and bring them in gradually...canned goods, toilet paper, etc. He asked if I had reached the point where I ran out to the trunk to tear off a few sheets of toilet paper when I had to go to the bathroom. The next step was for us to decide that I should feed the paper out through the trunk lid and just rip it off as needed!

NEVER VOLUNTEER
by Helen Rash

I told him I was supposed to wrap my arm with ACE bandages and try to keep it elevated as much as possible. He said, "Be careful...you might wind up volunteering for things you don't want!" ("Ladies and gentlemen, we have a buyer for the Van Gogh...sold to the lady with the bandages on her arm for four million dollars!")

RABBIT FOOD
by Rita Busch

Beta-carotene may help prevent some cancers, it is said. Therefore, we eat lots of carrot cake.

WATCH WHERE YOU STEP
by Rita Busch

As I was loading grocery bags in the car trunk, I felt something slide down my body and thought I'd dropped something. I looked down, and there was my silicone boob just lying there in the parking lot. I decided I'd rather not know if anyone had noticed, so without looking around, I picked it up, put it in a grocery bag and drove home, wondering if the cashier had noticed it starting to slide. I also bought new bras.

CONVERSATIONS
by Rita Busch

Rita and Daena:
Some doctors who don't do proper follow-up give cancer a bad name.
(Yeah, like it has a good name.)

* * * *

Tacked on to a House defense appropriations bill was funding for cancer research. Does that mean we'll get boobs instead of bombs?

* * * *

In "Monty Python and the Holy Grail," there's a scene where two knights are fighting in the woods. One keeps lopping off the other's limbs until there's nothing left but his torso and head. As I approached my second mastectomy (after years of chemo, TAXOL, baldness, etc.), I felt like that poor knight, who said, "Now I am *really* getting mad!"
(Helen)

* * * *

BJ asked Rita one day if she was going to have dessert. Rita said, "I'd love to, but I've eaten too much." BJ replied, "So have I, but I don't want to miss out on dessert." (BJ knew at the time she probably had only a few months to live.)

* * * *

Who, but a cancer survivor, would say—on being told she has tuberculosis—"Oh, Thank God! That's great news!"

* * * *

After a silicone implant: Remember the old ads for Toni home permanents? They showed twins with curly hair and asked, "Which twin has the Toni?" Now, I can say, "Which tit is the phony?"

A BARGAIN
by Rita Busch

One summer as I was walking to the cash register in Ross's, I saw a T-shirt in a purple and white abstract design on sale, so I picked it up without even trying it on. While cutting the labels off, I saw that the design would change color with body heat. One winter morning, I decided to wear the shirt when we went out for breakfast. After ordering breakfast, I was horrified to see that the entire shirt had turned pink except for the area around my implanted silicone breast! I rubbed on that area of the shirt to make it the same color as the rest of my shirt, and my husband pointed out that wasn't a real good thing to do in public. Great shirt sale.

EVERYTHING HAS ITS PLACE
by Rita Busch

Now that I have a prosthetic silicone breast, what do I do with it when undressing for a medical exam, X-ray, etc.? I've tried putting it in my purse, but there's no room. I've tried leaving it in my bra on a hanger, but the boob falls out. So, what are we to do? Make a space among the bandages and instruments on the only available flat surface and just plop it there?

DODGING, ARTFULLY
by Rita Busch

An art therapist came to our support group and asked us just to draw what we were feeling about cancer. I informed her that I had a little knowledge of art therapy, so perhaps it wouldn't work. She told me just to go ahead, anyway. While drawing what turned out to be a very angry picture, I leaned so hard on the red crayon that it broke and flew across the table. So much for my knowledge of art therapy interfering with the exercise.

CHAPTER SIX

Millions Of Us

BEAUTIFUL WOMEN
by Jana Morgana

Beautiful Women
Meeting in breast cancer support groups
Sharing hurts and successes
Relaxed Talking with women who know
Fear of having The Worst   Cancer
In charge or swept along
Choosing Doctors and procedures
Angry when not treated well
Feeling weak and out of control
Our Bodies have betrayed us
What did we do wrong
We cry   We have done the best we could
Love or hate for Siegel and Susan Love
Bodies in pain from Lumpectomy
Node Sampling Mastectomy Reconstruction
Tender   Spotted Tired from Radiation
Fatigue Nausea Wigs from Chemotherapy
Hot Flashes from Tamoxifen
Recovery Counting each Month Year
We let go of taking care of everyone

We listen and learn about ourselves
Beautiful Women
Knowing what we will do
With our lives

FAMILIAR REFRAIN
by Rita Busch

Heard in support groups round the world:
"I am really healthy—except for cancer, that is."

A CELEBRATION
by Lesley Tyson

a celebration of
camera happy coworkers
we need another picture
to be sure
for one revolutionary moment
the echo carries me back
to that day when the pictures
revealed the lump
that changed everything

ENCOUNTERING THE BEAST
by Daena Kluegel

These innocents, wandering carelessly, come upon a deep cave. Curious, they enter the dark cavern. While exploring, they travel further into the gloom and they discover a lump, a BEAST, in the dark cave interior. It is swollen, misshapen and virulently able to inflict vast misery.

There is no place to hide from the attack of the Beast. The innocents must do battle, fighting for survival while searching for a way out, back into the sunshine. Some get out with only a piece of themselves missing, slightly mutilated. Some never return from the dark, frightful interior, losing the battle. Some are dragged back again and again while fleeing the Beast, returning each time ravaged and diseased. None who have entered there are ever the same.

Helen, my dear, wonderful friend, you have been dragged back and savaged. How do we find and kill the BEAST without murdering ourselves? What talisman or magic medicine will protect us and our daughters?

HEALING
by Helen Rash

I awoke with four distinct images in my mind. Turning on the lamp, I took up the pen and pad of paper I'd left on the dresser the night before so I could record these. The plan was to fall asleep with Bob's wife on my mind and see if anything concerning her health came up overnight. Bob, a friend at work, and his wife were despairing that anyone would figure out why she had such severe pains in her abdomen. Twenty-five years earlier I'd learned to meditate; and one of the techniques we'd been taught was to project the mind to learn what might be troubling someone, even if we didn't know them. The next step was to send love and healing to the person. Bob had asked me to try this for his wife, whom I'd never met. The four pictures that came up were: the curve of a woman's back, which then became the curve of a banana; fingerlike growths similar to stalactites and stalagmites; and three evenly-spaced black dots, like the three holes in a bowling ball.

I'd also suggested that Bob and his wife go see my doctor, since I felt he was an excellent diagnostician. When I caught up with Bob two days later, he said my doctor had found undiagnosed scoliosis in his wife's spine. Also, some other doctor had recommended potassium supplements as a possible solution. I told Bob about the four images. I felt the curve of the back and the banana somehow related to what the two doctors had just said. That left two unexplained visions...the growths and the three holes.

I changed jobs, and a few months later Bob called me, his voice still reflecting amazement at what he was about to tell me. He said, "I just had to call you. You're not going to believe this." He went on to say that doctors had found that his wife's problem was a simple one...lesions in the form of "fingerlike growths" had resulted from an old appendectomy and were choking the intestine. They used a very modern laser technique to do non-invasive surgery on the lesions. When Bob's wife opened her gown to show him how they had gotten to her abdomen with the laser, all that remained were...three evenly-spaced holes.

I've always been fascinated that I can still use these techniques, even without any refresher training in the intervening years. Taking the Silva Method classes in 1972 was probably the single best decision I've ever made. We learned breathing, relaxation, guided imagery, and mind projection. These basic principles could then be used for problem-solving, such as stress and health management, habit control, improved memory, and relief from allergies. The instructor mentioned this last benefit just before I ended the classes and entered the fall hay fever season. My whole life I'd been plagued with severe allergies from mid-August to the first frost. I'd always gone out and gotten my prescription in August to get ready for the pollen. Without even trying any specific meditation focused on the allergies, I told myself that I wouldn't buy the drug...and that when the pollen entered my nose and eyes, my body would *not have* to react. An amazing thing happened that fall. I didn't have hay fever, and I haven't since. Had this been the *only* positive result of the Silva sessions, it still would have been worth the time and money I invested. To keep us grounded in reality, the teachers reminded us that we would continue to find hurdles in our lives...that daily meditation would not immunize us against difficulties but *would* help us deal with them. I've found this to be a very important part of learning to deal with problems. When, in my middle years, I was faced with chronic cancer, I became even bolder. As if I were the captain of a huge ship, I would "assemble" all the cells in my body and talk to them. Each cell was assigned a Teenage Mutant Ninja Turtle to protect it. I gave them a kind of Knute Rockne locker-room talk. "Now go out there and control any bad cells you find." I instructed them to whack the bad guys and dump them into my waste system.

Acupuncture

Meditation led me to explore other complementary forms of healing. In 1985, I heard a young man lecture on acupuncture and decided to go see him. We spent over an hour just talking about my medical history, family, and lifestyle. My dad, whom I'd loved very much, had died in 1977; and yet I still burst into tears randomly...especially when I tried to say the word "father." The acupuncturist didn't know this; and at one point I said to him, "I was very close to my..." and then began to sob. He said, "It's your father, isn't it? I knew it when you came through the door." What I found out later was that, in the five-element diagnosis technique of acupuncture, I am a "metal" person; and this is the element that includes the concept of "father." Thus, when I lost my dad, I was doubly hurt, because I felt a part of myself had been lost.

This first practitioner was moving away, so he gave me a letter of referral to the man I've been going to ever since. The referral letter suggested that Bob begin his treatments by focusing on my grief. Because the acupuncture was holistic, it dealt with restoration of harmony in the body, emotions, mind, and spirit.

The needles were very fine, not like hypodermic needles, and went in at a very shallow level. Sometimes I felt nothing, depending on how much imbalance there was in my body's energy. Other times there were various sensations...a dull ache or a kind of electrical flash. These were over very quickly, and even if he left the needles in place for a while, the discomfort was only momentary. Occasionally he would use cones of moxa, especially if I needed intense help. Moxa cones look like incense and give off a very pleasant aroma, or at least pleasant if one likes incense. Bob lit the tip of the cone and laid it at the same spot where a needle might have been used. When the skin felt very warm, I signaled him, and he removed it.

Going into acupuncture is really an act of faith, because the results of the treatments are not necessarily apparent immediately, although they can be. There have been many times when I became so relaxed during the treatment that I almost fell asleep on the table. There are no claims that acupuncture is a cure for severe problems such as advanced cancer, but it can strengthen the immune system and help with stress and other factors which could aggravate serious illness.

CAN YOU COME HERE WHERE I AM?

Psychics and Mediums

Because I'd frequently had psychic experiences through meditation, it was easy for me to believe that certain gifted people could be in touch with the Universal Spirit at an even stronger level and could offer insights. Through a Spiritualist Church in Georgetown I met two such women. My goal in meeting with them over the years has *not* been to get "advice" but to strengthen my belief in a higher power and the power of my own spirit. They have tapped into some amazing information over time; but two of the best examples related to my experience with the drug TAXOL and a woman I got to know when I was being treated with this anticancer drug.

"A Drug from the Bark of a Plant": In January of 1993, one of my psychics told me that I would have the opportunity to be treated with a drug that came from the bark of a plant and that this drug would be very good for me. This information had been passed to her by her spirit guide, an American Indian woman who'd been with her since childhood. The guide was "on the other side" (i.e., she was in spirit) and had access to universal intelligence. I was told this on a Saturday; and the next Thursday my oncologist informed me that he was considering putting me on TAXOL, which came from the bark of the yew tree. I gasped; but I didn't say anything to him, since he was skeptical of even basic alternatives, such as vitamin therapy.

"Elizabeth": When I went to the hospital for my second TAXOL dose, my roommate was a lovely woman who was also on her second dose, so we had something in common. She'd been battling ovarian cancer for six years, and TAXOL had been released to the public to fight this type of cancer. I was struggling with breast cancer, but my doctor felt the drug could help me also. In the short time we were together, I learned a lot about Elizabeth, her four young children, and her husband, whom I met.

Because we were both on a three-week treatment cycle, I was hoping we'd meet again...perhaps even share a room. My next dose had to be delayed a few days, but I did get to see her just before she checked out of the hospital and I checked in. Her husband was with her. She did not look good, as if she were losing the battle. She died shortly after that. The nurses on the ward told me, and I decided to write her husband a note. On a Friday he called me at work, and he spent a long time telling me how much he loved her and how he wouldn't have traded her for someone in perfect health. That night as I slept, I was overcome with a sense that Elizabeth knew he and I had talked. On Saturday I had an appointment with my psychic. She began by saying, "Before I begin your reading, I'd like to share with you that someone is here from spirit." She went on to say that this woman had died two months earlier (as had Elizabeth), and that the woman in spirit wanted to thank me for counseling recently with a member of her family. Ever since, I've felt a connection with this lovely woman from "the other side"…almost as if she were my guardian angel.

REMEDIES FOR RECOVERY
Daena Kluegel

Biofeedback has been around a long time but I had never paid much attention to it in spite of all the favorable articles I had read about it. When I came home from my surgery, a survivor took me to a Wellness Center for some workshops on nutrition and exercise. Mandy was very enthusiastic about the Center's biofeedback sessions and urged me to try it. "Well," I thought, "what have I got to lose? It may help with the anxiety and stress and even the aches and pains since I don't want to go through life on pain medication." Karen, the nurse practitioner and biofeedback counselor, was gentle and patient. She wired me up with little sensors which recorded stress in my face, shoulders, hands, and neck as I sat comfortably in a recliner chair. The first session was following a chemotherapy treatment and my readings even in the calm measurements were very high. The needles went off the grid on the chart for the stressors (hands in ice water, count out loud and backward by sevens for a minute and then visualize a situation which has made you very angry). She taught me relaxation techniques and how to read my own body's stress, and what kind of mental imagery and breathing helped. She taped her instructions and I had to practice it for twenty minutes twice a day. After six weeks, the charts were much more positive and I was often in the normal range without her cues.

I learned a lot from Biofeedback. I still practice the relaxation techniques. I have a mind/body imagery which I process through every morning when I wake up, right after my prayer of thanks for making it through another night safely. I have little A's and T's all over the interior of my body. They each have a sharp trident. They are marshaled out to find the malignant cells which I picture as black blobs. When one is found they stab it and kill it. Then all the black blobs are hoisted on the prongs of the trident and the A's and T's stuff those suckers down the sewer. Does it work? I don't know, but it does no harm and lets me attain a sense of control. It also helps take some of the edge off my anger. So I guess it does work for me.

I always thought of massage as a luxury for the well-off or athletes with injuries. After my surgery, I remembered that a friend had used therapeutic touch and massage to help regain flexibility and ease stiffness and pain in the node dissection arm. I called Nancy, a massage therapist in our church, and made an appointment. Nancy, a registered nurse, carefully checked my range of motion and listened to my complaints both physical and psychological. She felt that stress and anxiety increase discomfort and told me how I could help her help me while I was on the table. She started soft, soothing music playing and gave me imagery to focus on, a scene where I felt happy and calm, (I chose the beach). She held her hands about an inch over my body on the table and used them to "sense" the problem spots. She concentrated her firm yet gentle kneading and probing hands and fingers on those poor sore muscles. I usually fell asleep on the table wrapped in the warm blankets and comforted by Nancy's sure touch. She always ended by urging me to drink plenty of water to flush out the toxins. After I dressed, I felt light and relaxed and she sent me off with a warm smile and a hug.

During chemo, Nancy suggested using mental imagery to combat the nausea. She said blue was a very healing color. I remembered a chapel in Lucerne, Switzerland, where we saw beautiful Chagall windows of brilliant blue and yellow stained glass. I took that blue and made it surround and envelop me with clear light of that hue and intensity. It worked!

My oncologist was so supportive and understanding that when I told him how much therapeutic massage helped me with the side-effects of chemotherapy and the after-effects of the node dissection, he agreed to prescribe the therapy and the biofeedback sessions. His attitude was, "If it helps you get through the chemo treatment, then I want you to have it." He did not act as if I should just "get over it", and I am so grateful for his empathy. By prescribing the therapies, I was able to use my health insurance plan to defray part of the cost, which was a great help.

I have always taken vitamins, especially C, E and, after chemo, beta-carotene, which was recommended by a pharmacist. I then added selenium and calcium, (for my menopausal bones) and lecithin (for my short-term memory, recommended by an oncology nurse). I do not take inordinately large amounts, but I do take them daily. I increase the C if I have a cold beginning and it seems to help. I feel that they are fairly safe dietary supplements which may help my immune system (especially the antioxidants) even though there are conflicting studies on this. They cost a few dollars every month, but increase my feeling of doing what I can to stay healthy and disease free, so I think it is worth it. I know other survivors who have altered their lifestyles and diets or used other therapies. This works for me.

ELECTRIC ENERGY
by Lesley Tyson

electric energy
trapped on paper
trapped in our hearts
finding courage in community
to begin to decode
the uncomprehended message
stepping to the edge
to converge on the universal center
accepting the unchangeable
finding power within
to survive
to flourish
upon the acknowledgment
each day is a gift

FRIENDS
by Daena Kluegel and Helen Rash

HR: Daena is more than a fellow survivor. She is my good friend. We are a part of a little group of women I call "The Class of 1990." We went through the various phases of diagnosis and treatment at the same time, and this has created a bond which I think will last for many years. Two of our gang have moved far away, but we keep in touch. One of the group doesn't have a strong interest in the spiritual life, but she sends us love across the miles. Daena and I believe she *is* praying for us, even though our pal would never say the "P" word.

Recently I had to be admitted to the hospital by way of the Emergency Room. My crisis was not cancer-related, but I was very sick until they got me stabilized. I had IV tubes attached to my groin (the only place where they could find a vein quickly) and a tube down my nose and into my stomach. An orderly was wheeling me around the X-ray area when we ran right into Daena, who was there for an appointment. The orderly and I were chatting about which basketball team would win the NBA championship, when I heard Daena's familiar voice calling out to me. It was really good to see her.

She walked back to the ICU with us and spent some time at my bedside. We got into a discussion of something which struck us as funny, and I laughed till the tears rolled. I think the ICU nurse was not used to hearing raucous laughter from her patients. Daena knows how important it is for me to laugh, in spite of all we've been through. She also is very worried about me, although we don't say much about our fears. There are two kinds of panic when a friend gets cancer multiple times, as I have. I know Daena has been very sad and angry about my having to "return to battle" over and over; but I also know it must upset her deeply to think that this could happen to her. Often when she feels strongly about something, her cheeks turn very pink; and I see this when we talk about our common problem.

I've said almost daily that I don't know how I could have recovered and gotten on with life, had it not been for friends and family. My truest friends have known intuitively how to handle my crises. They know that the best thing they can do is just "be." That means having lunch with me, giggling over some inside joke, and letting me cry out loud. They also know that I'll give them a signal if I need help with groceries or feeding the cat. Daena understands this, and that's why we're such good friends.

DK: When a friend is diagnosed, you think about many things. It is always a sad time. So many thoughts go through your head. You want to spare a friend all the misery and agony but know there is only so much you can say or do. Still, if you've been there yourself, you can offer some things...advice, sympathy, support, listening. I will always be grateful to a survivor who got me out of my panic mode and into a doing mode by offering the advice, "Get to a teaching hospital."

When a survivor friend is diagnosed with a metastasis or recurrence, it is a very difficult time. Your first reaction is, "Oh no, she's been through enough, and why does it happen to a person who is so kind, sweet, and loving?" In Helen's case, she is all of these and more. She is an involved, active, and selfless woman with more courage than I've ever known. She is remarkable in her strength and resilience. Where I cry, she chooses laughter or song.

Then, you begin to think about what to do to help. What can you say to comfort? How can you "be there" for her? At the same time, this is another reminder and shock to you that, in spite of everything you may have done or changes you may have made to your lifestyle, you too are vulnerable to this same scenario.

I had to deal with that piece very quickly, as it was overwhelming me. It is hard to be a good friend in a panic. It is tempting to seek out escape or denial. But, the thought haunts me; can I stand it, the hurt of watching someone so vibrant suffer? I have done this twice before, and I do not know if I can go through it this time. I think of how scathing I've been regarding others who "dropped out" of Support Group or out of a

CAN YOU COME HERE WHERE I AM?

friendship during a crisis. I promised myself I would never desert...but how able am I? Can I watch, standing helplessly by, while that Beast devours what was Helen? Most of the time, I feel strong enough and trust that we who are her friends will find additional strength from each other if necessary.

Helen tries to spare us. She decides how much to put in each friend's hand. She considers our strengths and needs. Helen and I have made a bargain. We will talk about whatever needs to be talked about. We will try to be calm but realize that emotion is very near the surface. We will deal with and treat each new piece of information as we discover it. Helen gets to tell me when to panic, and only then will we panic. We will try to enjoy whatever else comes to us: laughter, movies, time to talk, and sharing our writing. I feel apprehensive that I'm not doing enough, but I wait for Helen to signal me about what she needs. She has been very specific about her fears about coping and her situation in a house with the bathroom and bedroom located upstairs. She also knows what she does not want or need right now...housecleaning services or people suggesting she's depressed. Helen is such a good and true friend, more like a sister, that I am willing to trust her and our bargain for now.

UNCERTAIN INITIATE
by Lesley Tyson

uncertain initiate
i did not expect to feel
such power
yet these spirits
burnished diamond bright
after their battles
with the enemy
offered an unconditional
sisterhood
and the life-force in that room
can last forever

SCHIZOID
by Rita Busch

I was not a good patient on chemotherapy. If my husband did some chore for me, I'd say, "Why are you doing that? I am not an invalid." If he didn't do a chore for me, I'd say, "I'm sick. How can you expect me to do that?"

SOMETIMES IT SEEMS
by Lesley Tyson

sometimes it seems as though
it was only a temporary phase
to have two breasts
i can no longer distinguish
between body deep memories
before and after
there is such clarity
in this present moment
it seems i was only waiting
to become this diamond bright creature
amazon
inevitable completion

ONE YEAR LATER
by Jana Morgana

One year after Breast Cancer at age 62
Dissatisfied   More than before
I'm still living alone   That hasn't changed
I have not put my images into a book
The Best New Thing
A writing Group walked in front of Me
I have written Prose Poems that satisfy
I hardly move   Sleeping is marvelous
I seldom want an adventure
Am I Different   I Am Different
I'm sorting down to the most
Fulfilling interactions with people
Sharing lives and feelings
Am I older and Bolder
And having more Fun than ever
Or sleep and cry and dream of
Having My Life more the Way I Want It
Have I done Enough
I'm Good Enough
I never Have to Do another thing
I'm Living My Life

SPARKLE
by Jana Morgana

Sun bursts of light
Bright and peaceful
Delightful   Content
Breathing
Exhilarated and calm
I am alright
For six months
I have been
Breathing carefully
Six months since
Breast Cancer surgery
Now sparkles are coming back

A REUNION OF BELLYDANCERS
by Helen Rash

I guess I've never been as physically fit as I was in my early thirties when I took four years of belly-dancing lessons. Really good Middle Eastern dance requires a lot of muscle control but also considerable flexibility. I learned to isolate my rib cage and move it separately from the rest of my body. I learned how to rotate my pelvis so that it *didn't* look like a stripper's routine. This distinction was really important to our teacher, who I'll call Jane. In those days D.C. had a number of good Greek and Middle Eastern restaurants with live music, and my friend Pat and I used to go out late Friday nights to see who was dancing where. I was fascinated as much by the spontaneous folk-dancing that whirled on the dance floor as I was by the people on stage. The men often got up and did wonderful primitive dance steps…very exciting. Sometimes Jane taught Pat and me some of the folk dances when she had time. After class the three of us would put on high black boots and, arms outstretched to each other's shoulders, we would dance the Sirtaki together.

Jane was probably in her late thirties, maybe older. We never knew. She had a wonderful, strong body, powerful legs and feet that gripped the floor when she danced barefoot, a lovely bosom that needed no support. She designed all her own costumes, beginning with a low-cut bra to which she sewed beads and sequins. She was the best belly-dancer I've ever seen. She was also the first woman I ever knew who had a mastectomy. In those days women signed waivers before surgery, allowing the doctor to decide whether to take the breast. She awoke to find the breast was gone. She handled things pretty well until she went looking for a prosthesis. Because most of them were not made with beautiful, young breasts as models, she literally beat her head against the wall of the dressing room in despair. But she was a strong-willed person; and she bounced back, redesigning all her outfits so that they draped over one shoulder in the style of ancient Greek gowns. She visited women in hospitals and spoke on local talk shows, and most importantly, she kept dancing.

Twenty years later, in 1993, she produced a "Gala Revue and Reunion," taking over the top floor of a restaurant and putting on a show of her students. I went, hoping to recapture some of the inspiration I'd always felt when I hung out at the Greek clubs.

There was some kind of county ordinance that forbid the showing of a woman's navel, and I was appalled by such Puritanism. That meant the dancers all had gauze film between their top and waist.

Jane had aged a great deal. Much about her face was the same, but her body was bloated and crippled with arthritis, and she had trouble walking. But the students who danced were very good and had learned a lot from her. When the show was over, the band played; and we got out on the floor and did some folk-dancing. This was wonderful. I had had my mastectomy two years before, but I shimmied and moved my shoulders just as if nothing had happened. I had not tried this for years, and I was, truly, inspired.

A GOOD YEAR
by Jana Morgana

I feel good about it
I have lived from 9 months to 21 months
After Breast Cancer surgery
I am still grumbling about
Not having my life the way I want it
I am a failure   Still no partner
I have a chronic pattern of dissatisfaction
In Reality Inside I am saying
Wow I want to celebrate
I smile and giggle   Life is OK
Maybe   I enjoy my life
This year I connected with
Starhawk's reclaiming collective
Affirmation   Magic   Power of Nature
During a weekend   For the first time
I felt Peacefully Satisfied with myself
During a week I celebrated and accepted
My fat and old body
On my twelfth trip to Hawaii
I felt Just Right   Being there
And was pleased with my two sons
Their wives and 10 grandchildren
I have changed

EXTINGUISHED CANDLES
by Lesley Tyson

extinguished candles
pictures of the wish
to reach the millennium
and beyond

AFTER THE FIRST INTIMATIONS
by Lesley Tyson

after the first intimations
of extinction
some by choice
test life's sweetness
with dangerous adventures
to reassert claims
to immortality
others by consequence
perform death-defying acts
and release eternity in trade
for the ability to savor
each present moment
quietly inventing
a new definition of courage

HAPPY BIRTHDAY, TO ME
by Katherine Traynham

Happy birthday, to me!
No more dread and consternation
No more counting of wrinkles, gray hairs and
Capped teeth, gingivitis and calcium hold no horror for me.
No more rubbing of broken veins and chubby ankles.
I'm a year older—whoopee! Happy birthday, to me!

Happy birthday, to me!
You think of face lifts, if you want
Of tummy-tucks to disguise yourself
And get a facial if it makes you feel better
Or refuse to tell your age and make us all guess
Hoping we'll miss by at least a decade.
I'm thrilled to be older—yahoo! Happy birthday, to me!

Happy birthday, to me!
I can't wait to see those jowly cheeks
Start to look like my grandmother's profile
Or get a little twinge of rheumatic in my shoulder
I'm hoping for dentures one day—or at least a partial plate

And no more hair dye for me until I need the one
That gives me that "blue" look I admire on other heads.

I can't wait, can't you see?
For someone small to call me Granny
Or my husband to tease we've been married "forever"
My children to chide, "Aren't you too old for that?"
To which I will gleefully chirp, YES! I AM too old for that
And getting older and older and older each year
Happy birthday, to me!

Go ahead and groan on your day
Tell the family to ignore it, you'd just as soon
Skip it, you're hating the thought of the numbers
That pile up, you're dreading the loss of your twentyish figure
You've worked awfully hard to pretend you're still 30
And I just can't wait to get older and older (I might not, you see)
So, happy birthday, to ME!

HOW BIG A DEAL IS IT
by Jana Morgana

I had Breast Cancer
0.5 centimeters 19 nodes negative
Lumpectomy   Radiation   No Drugs
Most likely   "This Cancer will never return"
I will not die from this Cancer
It's gone   Over   Is it a Big Deal
Am I Different
Eight Months after surgery
I have arm and breast pains
I feel emotions   Fear and cry more
I was angry at every inconvenience
Now I see mellowness
And peacefulness sweeping over me
Maybe I don't have to fight so hard
I use more of my time on what I want
I feel deeper connections
With loves   Friends   Nature   Me

HERE AND NOW
by Lesley Tyson

here and now on this crystal clear winter morning
with a sky so blue it brings tears to your eyes
i look back across the light years
since i first heard the word cancer
i can smile heart deep triumphant
at the memories of the living i have made since
from the beginning scheduling the mastectomy
so i could attend my only brother's wedding
i promised myself i would live each moment
to find something precious a heartbeat a spark
to reflect the grace and courage gifted to me
remembering that being here to feel
even the ache of a healing incision
even the aching emptiness after a lover's desertion
even the fear at the news of a recurrence
is still living
to call it only survival is too small a word
to know the intensity of
> the long frustrating days at work
> the pain of a twisted knee
> the task of changing a light bulb
> the sweet liquor of chocolate on the tongue
> the cutting icy winter air in the lungs
> the sticky humidity of a summer night
> the rainbow autumn in the mountains
> the crystal notes of a flamenco guitar
> the harmonies of voices singing chant
> the heartthrob purr of a small white cat
> the freedom of laughter
> the planning of something that matters
> the heart's slow unexpected reopening
> the splendor of sailing into venice at sunrise
it is all such sweet elixir
that i can perfect living forever in a single moment

ROLLER COASTER
by Rita Busch

I asked a kid on the bus to the Magic Kingdom which was the best ride and was told "Space Mountain," so Don and I headed straight there and got in the line which snaked around for about thirty minutes until we got near to the start of the ride and realized: 1) it was an indoor, dark roller coaster and roller coasters terrify me, and 2) we were the only adults in line except for a few who were accompanying children. Starting to do an about turn, I thought: I got through a cancer diagnosis and chemotherapy; I can surely get through a roller coaster ride.

I did. I hated it. I was terrified. I screamed every second. But you know, I felt good that I had done it. And I will never, ever, go on another roller coaster.

CRY ME A LIVER
by Katherine Traynham

Today, I danced naked through the bedroom. My children at college, my husband off to work, I was fresh from my bath and padding through to get to the closet. There, in front of the mirror, joy overtook me. I smiled at myself and nearly choked on giddiness.

So, I danced. I danced to "Only You," "Rock Around the Clock," and "R.E.S.P.E.C.T.," singing them myself, twirling my towel and cha-cha-ing until the expression on my dog's face told me I'd definitely gone too far. A chubby, graying, starting to wrinkle version of me, with dry skin and a belly and scars and cellulite, naked and playing alone in my bedroom!

Thank goodness no one saw me.

If only they could see me!

I wanted this, this living-thing, again. To be free of fear and hopelessness and be literally jumping for joy. I was only getting ready for work. Nothing spectacular happened to inspire me, except...

Except that I am happy. I had breast cancer, and I am still happy! Ain't that something? Despite the treatments, the depression, the abandonment of a few, the scars, the nagging feeling that I may yet have to meet this enemy on his own terms, the alone-ness of my own mortality—life is so deliciously good!

I have a body that doesn't work well anymore, but it stands me up in the morning and I can kiss my husband, let the dog out, hug my kids, write a letter. I can sing (not well, of course), play the piano, do embroidery, set the table, bake biscuits, visit a friend, answer the phones at work, file a deed, help a client, wrap a scarf around my neck instead of my head, feed the squirrels, polish the silver, call my sister, read the newspaper—jeez, I don't even have time in the day to do everything I can do that gives me pleasure.

I've buried friends and family and said good-bye to certain parts of me. I've cried a gallon of tears as if my life were the only important one in the world. I've been overtaken by medical

CAN YOU COME HERE WHERE I AM?

facts, been irritated at almost everyone, raged against the insensitive blobs, and guess what? Nothing killed it.

Nothing killed sweetness in life. Despite my best efforts to paint the world black, color bled through. The reddest cardinals sit and feed on my deck this gray winter. My husband bought me the bluest lapis lazuli earrings I've ever seen. The sun gets more gold every time I see it. My daughter's brown eyes have developed flecks of green in them. I started looking really good in deep, deep red. And after dancing naked, I stood in front of the mirror, thought about the months of chemo, and sang "Cry Me a *Liver*," wondering if anyone in the world could possibly be as funny as I am. Well, as funny as I *think* I am.

Garlic bread smells so good, I could inhale it. I am so good at embroidery now, everyone strokes the back of the napkins because they look as good as the front. The kids all bought me angels for the tree this Christmas because they are listening to me.

How could life be any better?

I have no idea how it happened.

There was no epiphany, no magic moment, no wise words from a stranger at the bus stop, no angelic trumpet, no majestic word from God, no sudden flash of light. Just the insistent, incessant creeping of life. Life that goes from one minute into the next, ready or not. Life that keeps living, regardless of circumstance or intent. One hair grew a millimeter, then the one next to it did. Cell by cell, the scar repaired the skin. A tenth of an ounce less tired today than yesterday. Two tears fewer each week. On a thousand-mile-walk, the first inch over with. Despite my best efforts, opening my eyes let something wonderful in. My daughters hugged each other in front of me. My husband laughed out loud at a joke. A Carolina chickadee sat still for a long moment right in front of my back door and let me see his face.

One bird. If there were only one bird in the world, I'd stay to try to see it. If there were one more question our daughters wanted to ask me, I'd want to hear it. If I can get one more stitch in on the part of the table runner that has the red berries,

I'll do it. One more Saturday to pick up the phone and hear my aunt's voice that sounds exactly like my mother's.

One more kiss from my beloved, courageous, handsome, generous, warrior husband. Even a little one.

Who could have such great, good, unexpected fortune? A friend who needs to talk to me, a warm fuzzy sweater, a dress-up party, the fattest cat I've ever seen.

I wouldn't miss it for the world.

Every second, something stunning happens. My house is beautiful to me. My grandmother's spoons need polishing and they feel wonderful in my hand. My sister gave me a box for photographs and it's wood and cherry stained! Isn't that the most wonderful thing you ever heard of?

I don't know what it is for you. I don't know if you have a friend, a husband, a child who can smile for you and give you a gift worth a treasure. I don't know if you have a squirrel in your backyard with brown ears and a torn-up tail who comes right up to the door when you forget to fill the feeder. I don't suppose everyone looks good in red.

But there's something. Something that will draw you back, even after breast cancer. Something that will make you hum to yourself. Some inexpressible thing of beauty, like a battered silver spoon a hundred years old. And that silly joy will come. Like a tiny chickadee in hesitation. Just one little bird of life. More powerful than cancer and far more intense than poison chemicals, it is. Life comes, more searing than radiation, sharper than any scalpel, pushing at you, insisting. It will drag you back, even when you're miserable. Like standing near an ocean, you'll be soaked in it soon. I don't know exactly what life is, but it's got its own agenda. If you're still breathing, it keeps tugging at you to get your attention. Molecules vibrate, the breeze shifts through a beech tree and, there you are. You felt wind on your face and liked it.

Kinda makes me want to dance naked! Or kiss a chickadee. Just one of them.

DON'T BE SURPRISED
by Judy Klevins and Helen Rash

Don't be surprised
>if you find yourself *taking* leave days for Caribbean snorkeling
>when you never before used vacation days.

Don't be surprised if you go on a date *rampage*
>putting ISO ads in the *"Washingtonian"*
>finding it's exhausting fun to have three dates in one day
>>and that *while* your sexual appetite may have been decreased
>>by Tamoxifen menopause
>your lust for life has raised your libido

Don't be surprised
>if it's suddenly easy to stay on a low-fat diet
>and lose those impossible pounds

Don't be surprised
>if the perfume you wore during chemo
>is no longer your favorite scent
>and you find new fragrances to take its place

Don't be surprised
>if you find yourself seeking gigglers and dreamers
>and avoiding whiners and dream-killers

Don't be surprised
>when the simple pleasures
>of a walk on a gray February morning
>or falling asleep with your lover
>or a slow-moving conversation
>with a high-school friend
>bring you to joyful tears

It's just life after cancer.

THREE WOMEN
by Jana Morgana

I have returned to Mother's hometown
To remember
I sit in the cemetery
Looking at the graves and cry
Feeling Mother-Elizabeth Jane
Grandmother-Teresa and Me
Holding hands in a circle
Crying and shaking together
Three women
We have done the best we could
Our lives are together forever
Now we can Love
And appreciate each other

COUNTING
by Lesley Tyson

counting

the rest of my lifetime
is counting...
one
start the cycle again
measuring my pulse
while i wait
for permission
for the examinations
to begin

...and counting
two
embracing myself
through the hospital gown
waiting
for the first answer
to develop
from those shadowed pictures
time stretches
i struggle to maintain hope
then they are before me
smiling
normal the excellent word
and i take a breath
move forward again

...and counting
three
the strong gentle fingers
deeply probe my scars
intensely searching my body
finding nothing

that does not belong
i take another
step forward

...and counting
four
my feet in the stirrups
as i learn
the periods are now
invisible
this chemical ending
is both hope and
protection
another step

...and counting
five
watching
with disconnected interest
as the stiletto steel fang
searches blindly for a vein
and the blue-red blood
to minutely reveal
any presence of the enemy
now wait through the days
for the answer

...and counting
six
reward
after impatient days
hear the word
normal
reprieve

WHO ARE THESE WOMEN, ANYWAY?

Daena Kluegel

Daena Kluegel has been married more than thirty years to a navy officer and computer analyst, is the mother of a talented architect son and gifted soprano daughter, a dedicated Montessori teacher, an amateur photographer, and a voracious reader. Life is very rich for her. Raised in the Midwest, Daena was an English major and found writing this book reawakened her long-dormant love of writing.

Daena was diagnosed in 1990 with intraductal carcinoma. A seven-year survivor now at fifty-five, she credits her mastectomy, chemotherapy, and alternative healing methods (biofeedback, therapeutic massage, prayer, support group, and the love of a good husband) for her recovery.

She'll tell you, "Cancer did not make me a better person," but if you push her, she'll admit it did "sharpen and focus" her. She's intent on fighting and living long enough to see breast cancer and its treatment a "plague of the past," like the polio epidemic of her childhood. In addition to her work with Breast Cancer survivor issues, she continues to take Spanish and writing classes and is constantly discovering new books to read, plays to see, and music to sing into the new century.

Kathe Traynham

Kathe Traynham grew up in the foothills of the Smoky Mountains in Tennessee, and so has a deep and abiding love for tall tales (lying) and storytelling. Naturally, she majored in English, but also Radio-TV-Film. A broadcast news producer in Memphis and New Orleans, she ended up in the Washington, D.C. area with ABC News' *World News Tonight with Peter Jennings*. In 1985, she married Peter Traynham, news photographer for CBS News and the love of her life. She continues a seven-generation tradition of women raising their own and others' children. Her family now includes a foster son, stepdaughter, and her biological daughter.

In 1995, at forty-four, she was diagnosed with breast cancer. She claims her years in television news prepared her for six months of chemotherapy and radiation treatment: producing network news pieces involves extreme fear, a belief that your life is at stake, nausea, and a certain amount of hair loss. In 1996, she completed Project LEAD, the National Breast Cancer Coalition's science course for breast cancer advocacy. She speaks to local groups about her experience with cancer and works to "stand in the gap" with newly diagnosed women in their shock.

In an effort to prove wrong those frustrated souls who declared her "unteachable," Kathe has now learned piano, embroidery, perfect baking-soda biscuits, and the alto parts to nearly every hymn written before 1920. For six years, she co-authored a weekly column called "Just As We Thought," which appeared in Northern Virginia newspapers. When in doubt, she resorts to quoting her mother—who really was always right.

Rita Busch

Rita Busch was eighteen and had seventy-five dollars when she left Scotland for Vancouver, British Columbia. She indulged her "wanderlust" for several years traveling, to Nassau, Quebec, Labrador, Grenada, Toronto, Labrador again, the UK again, and then, for a change of pace, settled in the Washington, D.C. area for twenty-seven years.

Rita was diagnosed with breast cancer in 1989. When it breached the chest wall in 1993, she was given three to five years to live. Since her current oncologist told her that was just an average, Rita claims (and we all agree) she's never been "average" about anything—and so she continues to ignore that prognosis.

In 1994, Rita moved with her husband to Las Cruces, New Mexico. Rita is witty and wry, and apparently, always tells the truth. We got something much better than great sweaters from Scotland: Rita and her "tumor humor."

Lesley Tyson

Don't try to figure out **Lesley Tyson**'s origins by her accent, or lack of one. She was born in Toronto, spent her childhood in upstate New York and "came of age" in Houston, Texas. The Virginia suburbs outside Washington were a compromise of climate, she says, somewhere between Toronto and Houston. Lesley works for a large government contractor. She joined the group not long after Rita left for New Mexico, and the project began to evolve into a book.

In 1991, she was diagnosed with systemic lupus erythematosus, which is now controlled with medication. Two years later, at age thirty-eight, a routine mammogram led to more tests and a breast cancer diagnosis. She then had a mastectomy and chemotherapy. A 1995 recurrence has responded well to further surgery, radiation, and Tamoxifen therapy.

Lesley is open, purposeful, vivacious, and tactful. Twenty-five years ago, her high school English teacher introduced his classes to free verse poetry and the precursor to today's "New Age" music. Since then, both have been an important part of Lesley's life. She uses her poetry as a healing tool and a celebration of life's "hopes, fears, triumphs, and uncertainties."

Jana Morgana

An artist in painting and assemblage, **Jana Morgana** also does land survey drafting. Born in 1933 in Wheeling, West Virginia, raised in Illinois, Missouri, and Utah, Jana then traveled to Stanford for her BA in Economics. Jana's four children have presented her with eleven grandchildren, so she's our official, reigning "Grandma" in the group. A twenty-seven-year marriage ended in divorce fourteen years ago.

In 1995, she was diagnosed with Stage I breast cancer and had a lumpectomy and radiation. Jana says she "never wrote anything" before joining our group. She claims the rest of us are "more verbal" than she is, but we suspect we're just louder. Jana describes her past year's accomplishments as "learning the habit of being satisfied with life."

She belongs to a colony of feminist artists, leads peer counseling support groups, works with incest survivors, and seeks out those who communicate through the spirit of nature. She brings a quiet examination of cancer and is passionate about giving women everywhere a voice for their experiences

Judy Thibault Klevins

Another native of Wheeling, West Virginia, **Judy Klevins** came to Virginia in 1967 to teach theater in Arlington Public Schools. After helping students create and present plays and television shows for twenty-eight years, she became the Arts Education Specialist for the system. Judy is our icon for romance after cancer. Following diagnosis and treatment, she met the right man and married him in 1996.

Judy discovered her Stage I breast cancer in 1992. A lumpectomy, radiation, Tamoxifen therapy, daily treats, massages, and other changes in lifestyle were her treatment choices.

She enjoys snorkeling, photography, and leading workshops at area universities. Although she will tell you she "came late to the group," we all remind her that she came just in time. We were assembling a manuscript when she added her work to ours. She's direct and helpful and hears rhythms in writing as well as theater and music.

Helen Rash

Helen Rash graduated from the University of Illinois with a B.S. in English, because the world can never have too many English majors! She taught school and managed human resources for the federal government until her early retirement. Since then, she wanted to spend as much time as possible "living in the right side of her brain," painting, writing, and enjoying friends. She also volunteered in fellow writer Daena Kluegel's Montessori classroom and at the Center for Mind-Body Medicine.

When we started writing, Helen had already lived with cancer longer than any of us. She was diagnosed in 1966 with ovarian cancer. She was only twenty-five. Helen said she must have been too young to quite understand how unlikely it was that she would survive that cancer for more than twenty-five years. Helen began her "long and illuminating journey with breast cancer" in 1989.

We are all still entranced with Helen's stories about her belly dancing lessons, modeling, and singing. (Her telephone answering machine featured her singing something from the '40's or earlier—and she was good!) Helen was single and we encouraged her to write her version of "The Rules: Dating Tips for Mammary-Challenged Women."

Helen died just as summer began, 1997. This book, which she was so sure would be published, was one of the last things she talked about just two days before she died. She was smiling, naturally.